Cases for PACES

Cases for PACES

Stephen Hoole
Consultant Cardiologist
Royal Papworth Hospital
Cambridge, UK

Andrew Fry
Consultant in Acute Medicine and Nephrology
Addenbrooke's Hospital
Cambridge, UK

Rachel Davies
Consultant Respiratory Physician
Hammersmith Hospital
London, UK

Fourth Edition

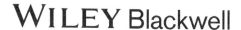

This fourth edition first published 2025
© 2025 by John Wiley & Sons Ltd

Edition History
Stephen Hoole, Andrew Fry, Daniel Hodson & Rachel Davies (1e, 2003 and 2e, 2010); John Wiley &
Sons Ltd (3e, 2015)

Registered Offices
John Wiley & Sons, Inc., 111 River Street, Hoboken, NJ 07030, USA
John Wiley & Sons Ltd, The Atrium, Southern Gate, Chichester, West Sussex, PO19 8SQ, UK

For details of our global editorial offices, customer services, and more information about Wiley products
visit us at www.wiley.com.

Wiley also publishes its books in a variety of electronic formats and by print-on-demand. Some content
that appears in standard print versions of this book may not be available in other formats.

Library of Congress Cataloging-in-Publication Data applied for
Paperback ISBN: 9781119576501

Cover Design: Wiley
Cover Image: © Kreativorks/iStock/Getty Images

Set in 7.5/9.5pt Frutiger by Straive, Pondicherry, India

SKY10081218_080624

Contents

Foreword, ix
Preface, x
Acknowledgements, xii
Abbreviations, xiii
Advice, xx

Respiratory, 1

Clinical mark sheet, 1
Respiratory exam – general advice, 2
Pulmonary fibrosis, 4
Bronchiectasis, 5
Old tuberculosis, 6
Surgical respiratory cases, 7
Chronic obstructive airways disease, 8
Pleural effusion, 10
Lung cancer, 12
Cystic fibrosis, 14
Pneumonia, 15
Pulmonary hypertension, 17

Cardiology, 19

Clinical mark sheet, 19
Cardiology exam – general advice, 20
Aortic stenosis, 22
Aortic incompetence, 25
Mitral stenosis, 27
Mitral incompetence, 29
Tricuspid incompetence, 31
Pulmonary stenosis, 32
Prosthetic valves: aortic and mitral, 33
Implantable devices, 35
Constrictive pericarditis, 36
COMMON CONGENITAL DEFECTS, 38
Atrial septal defect, 38
Ventricular septal defect, 39
ASSOCIATIONS WITH CONGENITAL VSD, 40
1. Fallot's tetralogy, 40
2. Coarctation, 40
3. Patent ductus arteriosus (PDA), 40
Hypertrophic (obstructive) cardiomyopathy, 42
Heart failure, 44

Neurology, 46

Clinical mark sheet, 46
Neurology exam – general advice, 47
Dystrophia myotonica, 51
Cerebellar syndrome, 53
Multiple sclerosis, 54
Stroke, 56
Spastic legs (i.e. spinal cord lesion), 59
Syringomyelia, 61
Motor neurone disease, 63
Parkinson's disease, 64
Hereditary motor sensory neuropathy
aka Charcot–Marie–Tooth, 66
Friedreich's ataxia, 67
Facial weakness, 68
Myasthenia gravis, 70
Tuberous sclerosis, 71
Neurofibromatosis, 72
Abnormal pupils, 73
Horner's pupil, 73
Holmes–Adie (myotonic) pupil, 73
Argyll Robertson pupil, 74
Oculomotor (III) nerve palsy, 74
Optic atrophy, 75
RETINAL PATHOLOGY, 77
Age-related macular degeneration, 77
Retinitis pigmentosa, 78
Retinal artery occlusion, 79
Retinal vein occlusion, 79

Abdominal, 80

Clinical mark sheet, 80
Abdominal exam – general advice, 81
Chronic liver disease and hepatomegaly, 83
Haemochromatosis, 86
Splenomegaly, 88
Renal enlargement, 90
The liver transplant patient, 92
The renal patient, 93

Communication, 95

Clinical mark sheet, 95
Communication station – general advice, 96
ETHICS AND LAW IN MEDICINE, 97

Principles of medical ethics, 97
Competency and consent, 98
Legal aspects, 98
Confidentiality, 101
End-of-life decisions, 102
TYPES OF COMMUNICATION, 104
Information delivery, 104
Breaking bad news, 105
Dealing with a difficult patient, 106
WORKED EXAMPLES, 108
Duty of candour/medical mistake, 108
Advanced care planning, 108
Needlestick injury, 110
Epilepsy, 111
Huntington's chorea, 111
Paracetamol overdose, 112
Brain-stem death and organ donation, 113
Non-compliant diabetic, 115
Vaccination compliance, 116
Shared decision making, 117
Sample questions for self-directed learning, 119

Consultations, 120
Clinical mark sheet, 120
Consultation – general advice, 121
Chest pain, 122
Pericarditis with effusion, 124
Atrial fibrillation, 125
Hypertension, 127
Eisenmenger's syndrome, 130
Ataxia, 131
Headache, 132
Altered conscious state, 135
Syncope, 137
Worsening mobility, 139
Fall and a fragility fracture, 141
Dyspnoea – asthma, 142
Dyspnoea – acute pulmonary embolus, 144
Haemoptysis, 146
Persistent fever, 148
Anaemia, 151
Sickle cell disease, 153
Glandular fever, 155
Nephrotic syndrome, 157

Jaundice, 159
Inflammatory bowel disease, 161
Infectious (traveller's) diarrhoea, 164
Swollen calf, 166
Leg ulcers, 168
Red rashes, 170
Skin malignancy, 174
Skin and hyperextensible joints, 176
Rheumatoid arthritis, 178
Systemic lupus erythematosus, 181
Systemic sclerosis, 183
Ankylosing spondylitis, 185
Marfan's syndrome, 186
Paget's disease, 188
Other joint problems, 189
Hypercalcaemia, 191
Diabetes and complications, 192
General diabetes questions, 192
Diabetes and the skin, 192
Diabetic retinopathy, 194
Hyperthyroidism and Graves' disease, 197
Hypothyroidism, 199
Amenorrhoea, 201
Acromegaly, 203
Cushing's syndrome, 205
Addison's disease, 208

Index, 210

Foreword

Taking the MRCP PACES exam is a defining moment in most physicians' training life. PACES is undoubtedly a high-stakes exam both from the perspective of the implications for progression of training but also for the way an individual's knowledge and skills are placed under the spotlight. All physicians will have strong memories of their PACES experience; both good and bad. It is a stern test, but once completed it acts as a stamp of quality that is indelible and widely recognized. Getting through the exam successfully requires hard work, dedication and a pragmatic approach given the competing pressures of both clinical and home life.

This book can't replace hard work and dedication, but it does provide a well-proven and effective methodology for success. Thousands of physicians have benefited from the use of its wisdom and the fact it is now in its fourth generation is testament to how useful it has been for many. This latest edition takes into account the evolving design of the exam and should lessen the fear of the unknown that some have when approaching the exam. PACES will continue to evolve as medicine itself evolves, but it is striking how much the principles of clinical diagnosis remain constant. The advice to take time to think, look and gather oneself while the hand rub dries is one such principle. These principles are not just for the exam but when used in daily clinical practice will make life simpler and less stressful for the physician and result in better outcomes for the patient.

The breadth of internal medicine is wide and this book reminds us how much we have learned (or indeed still have to learn or relearn). It reminds us how fascinating medicine is and why many of us have chosen life as a physician – and given current clinical pressures such a reminder is always helpful. For those taking the exam, you will never again have such a wide breadth of knowledge and hopefully this book will help you keep much of that accumulated wisdom for all your professional life.

I wish you all the best for the exam and hope this book eases the journey through it. I suspect it will and if you have a hard copy you will keep it to refer to for many years to come. You may even read these words again in 20 years' time (he says as he looks at the dog-eared spine of the copy of its predecessor on the office shelf!).

Prof. Andrew Goddard
Consultant Gastroenterologist, Royal Derby Hospital
Past President of the Royal College of Physicians, London

Preface

PACES (Practical Assessment of Clinical Examination Skills) was initiated in June 2001 by the Royal College of Physicians as the final stage of the MRCP examination. The initial examination consisted of five stations in a carousel: Station 1: Respiratory/Abdominal (10 minutes each), Station 2: History Taking (20 minutes), Station 3: Cardiology/Neurology (10 minutes each), Station 4: Communication Skills and Ethics (20 minutes) and Station 5: Short Cases (Skin, Locomotor, Eyes and Endocrine: 5 minutes each). The format was refined in October 2009 by restructuring Station 5 into two 10-minute 'Brief Clinical Consultations'.

The PACES exam had a further major update introduced from Autumn 2023 that was badged PACES23. Many aspects of the exam remain the same as the old format and the standard required to pass PACES23 is also unchanged. There will still be a five-station carousel, with each station lasting 20 minutes and 5-minute intervals in between. Candidates will continue to be examined by two examiners, who will have calibrated the case and agreed the pass threshold before assessing and marking each candidate independently.

The assessment of seven key skills is also retained in PACES23:

A. Physical Examination
B. Identifying Clinical Signs
C. Communication
D. Differential Diagnosis
E. Clinical Judgement
F. Managing Patient Concerns
G. Maintaining Patient Welfare

Candidates must achieve a pass in all seven key skills and reach a total mark above a set threshold to pass.

The four clinical encounters assessing Respiratory, Abdominal, Cardiovascular and Neurological systems, each in 10 minutes, with 6 minutes to examine and 4 minutes to interact with examiners, also remain the same. However, Station 2 – History Taking without physical examination was thought to be unrepresentative of current clinical practice and has been removed; Station 4 – Communication was believed to be too long, with examiner interaction of little value in assessing the candidate; and Station 5 – Brief Clinical Consultations was too short, although this station provided the best integrated assessment of all seven key skills that emulated real-life clinical practice. Stations 4 and 5 have now been redesigned, with more emphasis on the clinical consultation:

Old MRCP PACES		New PACES23
Station 2 – 20-min History Taking	→	Removed
Station 4 – 20-min Communication	→	2 × 10-min Communication encounter without examiner interaction
Station 5 – 2 × 10-min Brief Clinical Consultation	→	2 × 20-min Consultations: 15 minutes history and examination and 5 minutes examiner interaction

The five-station carousel has also been redesigned to accommodate these changes, with the two Communication encounters preceding the Respiratory encounter in Station 1 and Abdominal encounter in Station 4, two Consultation encounters (Station 2 and 5) and the Cardiovascular and Neurology encounters in Station 3 remaining unchanged:

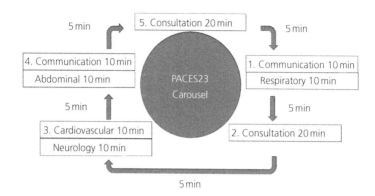

Cases for PACES Fourth Edition prepares candidates for the current PACES23 examination. It mimics the new examination format and is designed for use in an interactive way. This fourth edition has a completely revised text that has been informed by recent successful candidate feedback. It has useful advice for the day of the exam and provides updated information on clinical, ethical and medicolegal issues. There are plenty of new scenarios and mock questions for candidates to practise themselves. The two Consultation stations, which assess all seven key skills in an integrated way that most closely reflects day-to-day practice, account for two-fifths of the exam marks and receive particular attention in this new edition.

Avoid further factual cramming at this stage – you know enough! Go and see medical patients on a busy acute medicine unit or outpatient department. This has always been the best way to prepare for PACES and will be particularly beneficial for the new Consultation stations. This book will assist you in self-directed ward revision in preparation for PACES23. Each section has clinical mark sheets guiding which of the seven skills are being assessed and what you need to demonstrate to pass; this should enable groups of candidates to practise 'under examination conditions' at the bedside.

Common cases that regularly appear in the exam, rather than rarities, have been deliberately chosen. We assume candidates who are well practised will be fluent in the examination techniques needed to elicit the various clinical signs. However, in this new edition we provide extra guidance on how to efficiently examine each system to identify and interpret those all-important clinical signs within the allotted time.

We provide discussion topics that a candidate could be expected to comment on at the end of the case during the 4 or 5 minutes of examiner interaction. Remember that the examiners are specifically assessing your knowledge of the differential diagnosis and organized clinical judgement and management, while addressing the patient's concerns and maintaining patient welfare throughout this interaction.

The detail in this book is not exhaustive but rather what is reasonably needed to pass and be a competent and safe Specialty Registrar practising medicine with minimal supervision. There is space to make further notes if you wish. The aim of this book is to put the information that is frequently tested in the clinical PACES23 examination in a succinct, exam-style format that will enable capable candidates to practise and pass with ease on the day.

We wish you the best of luck.

Stephen Hoole
Andrew Fry
Rachel Davies

Acknowledgements

We acknowledge the help of Dr Daniel Hodson in the first and second editions, Dr William Brown for his assistance in updating the neurology station and Dr Peter Scanlon for his advice on the retinopathy cases. We thank the doctors who taught us for our own PACES examination, and above all the patients who allow us to refine our examination techniques and teach the next generation of MRCP PACES candidates.

Abbreviations

AAA	Abdominal aortic aneurysm
ABC	Airway, breathing, circulation
ABG	Arterial blood gas
ABPA	Allergic bronchopulmonary aspergillosis
ABPM	Ambulatory blood pressure monitoring
ACE	Angiotensin-converting enzyme
ACh	Acetylcholine
AChR	Acetylcholine receptor
ACR	Albumin: creatinine ratio
ACS	Acute coronary syndrome
ACTH	Adrenocorticotrophic hormone
ADLs	Activities of daily living
ADPKD	Autosomal dominant polycystic kidney disease
ADRT	Advanced decisions to refuse treatment
AF	Atrial fibrillation
AFB	Acid-fast bacillus
AFP	Alpha-fetoprotein
AICD	Automated implantable cardiac defibrillator
AIDP	Acute inflammatory demyelinating polyradiculoneuropathy
AIH	Autoimmune hepatitis
A(I)NOCA	Angina (ischaemia) non-obstructive coronary artery
AKI	Acute kidney injury
ALP	Alkaline phosphatase
AMD	Age-related macular degeneration
ANA	Anti-nuclear antibody
APS	Anti-phospholipid syndrome
AR	Aortic regurgitation
ARB	Angiotensin II receptor blocker
ARNI	Angiotensin receptor/neprilysin inhibitor
ARVD	Arrhythmogenic right ventricular dysplasia
AS	Aortic stenosis
5-ASA	5-Aminosalicylic acid
ASD	Atrial septal defect
ASOT	Anti-streptolysin O titre
ATP	Anti-tachycardia pacing
AV	Arteriovenous
AVN	Atrioventricular node
AVR	Aortic valve replacement
AVSD	Atrioventricular septal defect
AXR	Abdominal X-ray
BAV	Balloon aortic valvuloplasty
BFT	Bone function test
BIPAP	Bi-level positive airway pressure
BiV	Biventricular
BM	Boehringer Mannheim (glucose)
BMI	Body mass index
BNF	British National Formulary
BNP	Brain natriuretic peptide
BP	Blood pressure
BPA	Balloon pulmonary angioplasty

BPPV	Benign paroxysmal positional vertigo
BSO	Bilateral salpingo-oophorectomy
BT shunt	Blalock–Taussig shunt
CA	Carcinoma
CABG	Coronary artery bypass graft
CAD	Coronary artery disease
CAP	Community-acquired pneumonia
CAPD	Continuous ambulatory peritoneal dialysis
CCB	Calcium channel blocker
CCF	Congestive cardiac failure
CCP	Cyclic citrullinated peptide
CF	Cystic fibrosis
CFA	Cryptogenic fibrosing alveolitis
CFTR	Cystic fibrosis transmembrane conductance regulator
CGM	Continuous glucose monitor
CGRP	Calcitonin gene-related peptide
CIDP	Chronic inflammatory demyelinating polyneuropathy
CK	Creatine kinase
CKD	Chronic kidney disease
CLD	Chronic liver disease
CMD	Coronary microcirculatory dysfunction
CML	Chronic myeloid leukaemia
CMR	Cardiovascular magnetic resonance
CMV	Cytomegalovirus
CNS	Central nervous system
CoA	Coarctation of aorta
COPD	Chronic obstructive pulmonary disease
COMT	Catechol-o-methyl transferase
CPET	Cardiopulmonary exercise test
CRP	C-reactive protein
CRT	Cardiac resynchronization therapy
CRT-D	Cardiac resynchronization therapy defibrillator
CSF	Cerebrospinal fluid
CT	Computed tomography
CTCA	CT coronary angiography
CTEPH	Chronic thromboembolic pulmonary hypertension
CTPA	CT pulmonary angiography
CV	Cardiovascular
CVA	Cerebrovascular accident
CVID	Common variable immunodeficiency
CVS	Cardiovascular system
CXR	Chest X-ray (radiograph)
DBD	Donation after brain death
DBP	Diastolic blood pressure
DCD	Donation after cardiac death
DIOS	Distal intestinal obstruction syndrome
DIPJ	Distal interphalangeal joint
DKA	Diabetic ketoacidosis
DM	Diabetes mellitus
DM1	Dystrophia myotonica type 1
DM2	Dystrophia myotonica type 2
DMARD	Disease-modifying anti-rheumatic drug
DNA-CPR	Do not attempt cardiopulmonary resuscitation
DNAR	Do not attempt resuscitation

DNase	Deoxyribonucleic acid hydrolytic enzyme
DOAC	Direct oral anticoagulant
D&V	Diarrhoea and vomiting
DVLA	Driver and Vehicle Licensing Agency
DVT	Deep vein thrombosis
eGFR	Estimated glomerular filtration rate
EBUS	Endobronchial ultrasound
EBV	Epstein–Barr virus
EC	Ejection click
ECG	Electrocardiogram
ECHO	Echocardiogram
EEG	Electroencephalogram
EF	Ejection fraction
EMG	Electromyogram
EP	Electrophysiology
ERA	Endothelin receptor antagonist
ERCP	Endoscopic retrograde cholangiopancreatography
ESM	Ejection systolic murmur
ESR	Erythrocyte sedimentation rate
EtOH	Ethanol
ETT	Exercise treadmill test
EVAR	Endovascular aortic repair
FBC	Full blood count
FEV$_1$	Forced expiratory volume in 1 second
FFP	Fresh frozen plasma
FH	Family history
FSGS	Focal segmental glomerulosclerosis
FSH	Follicle-stimulating hormone
FSHD	Facioscapulohumeral muscular dystrophy
FTA	Fluorescent treponema antibodies
FVC	Forced vital capacity
GA	General anaesthetic
GBS	Guillain–Barré syndrome
GCS	Glasgow Coma Scale
GEP	Gastro-entero-pancreatic
GGT	Gamma-glutamyl transferase
GH	Growth hormone
GI	Gastrointestinal
GLP-1	Glucagon-like peptide-1
GMP	Good medical practice
GnRH	Gonadotropin-releasing hormone
GORD	Gastro-oesophageal reflux disease
Gp	Glycoprotein
GRACE	Global Registry of Acute Coronary Events
GTN	Glyceryl trinitrate
Hb	Haemoglobin
HBPM	Home blood pressure monitoring
HBV	Hepatitis B virus
HCC	Hepatocellular carcinoma
HCG	Human chorionic gonadotrophin
HCM	Hypertrophic cardiomyopathy
HCV	Hepatitis C virus
HDU	High-dependency unit
HF	Heart failure

HGV	Heavy goods vehicle
HIV	Human immunodeficiency virus
HLA	Human lymphocyte antigen
HOCM	Hypertrophic obstructive cardiomyopathy
HR	Heart rate
HRT	Hormone replacement therapy
HSMN	Hereditary sensory motor neuropathy
HSV	Herpes simplex virus
5-HT	5-hydroxytryptamine
IABP	Intra-aortic balloon pump
IBD	Inflammatory bowel disease
ICD	Implantable cardioverter defibrillator
IDDM	Insulin-dependent diabetes mellitus
IGF	Insulin-like growth factor
IHD	Ischaemic heart disease
ILD	Interstitial lung disease
INR	International normalized ratio
IPF	Idiopathic pulmonary fibrosis
IRMA	Intraretinal microvascular abnormalities
ITP	Immune thrombocytopenic purpura
ITU	Intensive therapy unit
IV	Intravenous
IVC	Inferior vena cava
IVDA	Intravenous drug abuse
JVP	Jugular venous pressure
K$_{co}$	Transfer coefficient
LA	Left atrial
LAA	Left atrial appendage
LAAO	Left atrial appendage occlusion
LACS	Lacunar anterior circulation stroke
LAD	Left axis deviation
LDH	Lactate dehydrogenase
LEMS	Lambert–Eaton myasthenic syndrome
LFT	Liver function test
LGE	Late gadolinium enhancement
LH	Luteinizing hormone
LMN	Lower motor neurone
LMWH	Low molecular weight heparin
LP	Lumbar puncture
LQTS	Long QT syndrome
LRTI	Lower respiratory tract infection
LTOT	Long-term oxygen therapy
LTR	Left to right
LV	Left ventricle
LVAD	Left ventricular assist device
LVEDP	Left ventricular end-diastolic pressure
LVEF	Left ventricular ejection fraction
LVH	Left ventricular hypertrophy
LVOT	Left ventricular outflow tract
mAb	Monoclonal antibody
MAO	Monoamine oxidase
MCPJ	Metacarpophalangeal joint
MC + S	Microscopy, culture and sensitivity
MDM	Mid-diastolic murmur

MDT	Multi-disciplinary team
MEN	Multiple endocrine neoplasia
MG	Myasthenia gravis
MI	Myocardial infarction
MIBI	Myocardial perfusion (sestamibi) imaging
MLF	Medial longitudinal fasciculus
MMF	Mycophenolate mofetil
MND	Motor neurone disease
mPAP	Mean pulmonary artery pressure
MPTP	Methyl-phenyl-tetrahydropyridine
MR	Mitral regurgitation
MRA	Magnetic resonance angiography
MRCP	Magnetic resonance cholangiopancreatography
MRI	Magnetic resonance imaging
MS	Mitral stenosis
MSA	Multisystem atrophy
MTPJ	Metatarsophalangeal joint
MuSK	Muscle-specific kinase
MV	Mitral valve
MVP	Mitral valve prolapse
MVR	Mitral valve replacement
6MWD	Six-minute walk distance
NG	Nasogastric
NHSE	NHS England
NIPPV	Non-invasive positive pressure ventilation
NOAC	Non-vitamin K antagonist oral anticoagulant
NSAID	Non-steroidal anti-inflammatory drug
NSCLC	Non-small cell lung cancer
NT-proBNP	N-terminal prohormone of brain natriuretic peptide
NVD	Neovascularization of the disc
NVE	New vessels elsewhere
NYHA	New York Heart Association
OA	Osteoarthritis
OAC	Oral anticoagulant
OCP	Oral contraceptive pill
OGD	Oesophago-gastro-duodenoscopy
OS	Opening snap
Pa	Partial pressure (arterial)
PACS	Partial anterior circulation stroke
PAH	Pulmonary arterial hypertension
PBC	Primary biliary cirrhosis
PCOS	Polycystic ovary syndrome
PCR	Polymerase chain reaction
PCT	Primary Care Trust
PCWP	Pulmonary capillary wedge pressure
PD	Parkinson's disease
PDA	Patent ductus arteriosus
PDE5	Phosphodiesterase-5
PE	Pulmonary embolism
PEA	Pulmonary endarterectomy
PEFR	Peak expiratory flow rate
PEG	Percutaneous endoscopic gastrostomy
PEP	Post-exposure prophylaxis
PET	Positron emission tomography

PH	Pulmonary hypertension
PICA	Posterior inferior cerebellar artery
PIPJ	Proximal interphalangeal joint
PLA2R	Anti-phospholipase A2 receptor
PMH	Past medical history
PMR	Polymyalgia rheumatica
PPCI	Primary percutaneous coronary intervention
PPI	Proton pump inhibitor
PPMS	Primary progressive multiple sclerosis
PPRF	Paramedian pontine reticular formation
PPVI	Percutaneous pulmonary valve implantation
PR	Per rectum (rectal)
PRL	Prolactin
PRN	*Pro re nata*, when required
PS	Pulmonic stenosis
PSA	Prostate specific antigen
PSC	Primary sclerosing cholangitis
PSM	Pan-systolic murmur
PSV	Public service vehicle
PTH	Parathyroid hormone
PTHrP	Parathyroid hormone-related peptide
PUVA	Psoralen ultraviolet A
PV	*Per vaginum* (vaginal)
PVD	Peripheral vascular disease
PVR	Pulmonary vascular resistance
QoL	Quality of life
RA	Rheumatoid arthritis
RAD	Right axis deviation
RADT	Rapid antigen detection test
RAPD	Relative afferent pupillary defect
RAS	Renal artery stenosis
RAST	Radio-allergo-sorbent test
RBBB	Right bundle branch block
RCC	Right coronary cusp
RF	Risk factor
RR	Respiratory rate
RRMS	Relapsing-remitting multiple sclerosis
RTL	Right to left
RUQ	Right upper quadrant
RV	Right ventricle
RVF	Right ventricular failure
RVH	Right ventricular hypertrophy
Rx	Treatment
SAH	Subarachnoid haemorrhage
sAVR	Surgical aortic valve replacement
SBP	Systolic blood pressure
SCD	Sudden cardiac death
SCLC	Small cell lung cancer
SGLT2	Sodium-glucose co-transporter 2
SH	Social history
SIADH	Syndrome of inappropriate anti-diuretic hormone
S-ICD	Subcutaneous implantable cardiac defibrillator
SLE	Systemic lupus erythematosus
SOA	Swelling of ankles

SOB	Shortness of breath
SOL	Space-occupying lesion
SPMS	Secondary progressive multiple sclerosis
SSRI	Selective serotonin reuptake inhibitor
SVCO	Superior vena cava obstruction
SVT	Supraventricular tachycardia
T$_4$	Thyroxine
T°C	Temperature
TACS	Total anterior circulation stroke
TAVI	Transcutaneous aortic valve implantation
TB	Tuberculosis
TEER	Transcatheter edge-to-edge repair
TENS	Transcutaneous electrical nerve stimulation
TFT	Thyroid function test
THR	Total hip replacement
TIA	Transient ischaemic attack
TIMI	Thrombolysis in myocardial infarction
TKI	Tyrosine kinase inhibitor
TLC	Total lung capacity
TL$_{co}$	Carbon monoxide transfer factor
TNM	Tumour nodes metastasis (staging)
TOE	Transoesophageal echo
ToF	Tetralogy of Fallot
tPA	Tissue plasminogen activator (alteplase)
TPHA	Treponema pallidum haemagglutination assay
TPMT	Thiopurine methyltransferase
TPW	Temporary pacing wire
TR	Tricuspid regurgitation
TSAT	Transferrin saturation
TSH	Thyroid stimulating hormone
TTE	Transthoracic echo
tTG	Tissue transglutaminase
TTR	Time in therapeutic range
TV-ICD	Transvenous implantable cardiac defibrillator
TWI	T-wave inversion
U&E	Urea and electrolytes
uACR	Urine albumin: creatinine ratio
UC	Ulcerative colitis
UFH	Unfractionated heparin
UIP	Usual interstitial pneumonia
UKHSA	UK Health Security Agency
UMN	Upper motor neurone
uPCR	Urine protein: creatinine ratio
US	Ultrasound
UTI	Urinary tract infection
VATS	Video-assisted thoracoscopic surgery
VEGF	Vascular endothelial growth factor
VEP	Visual evoked potential
VIP	Vasoactive intestinal peptide
VQ	Ventilation–perfusion
VSD	Ventricular septal defect
VT	Ventricular tachycardia
VTE	Venous thromboembolism
WCC	White cell count

Advice

Preparation

Practice makes perfect: it makes the art of eliciting clinical signs second nature and allows you to concentrate on what the physical signs actually mean. Practice makes you fluent and professional and this will give you confidence under pressure. We strongly encourage you to see as many patients as possible in the weeks leading up to the exam. Practise under exam conditions with your peers, taking it in turns to be the examiner, and use the mark sheets provided. This is often very instructive and an occasionally amusing way to revise! It also maintains your motivation as you see your performance improve. We encourage you to seek as much help as possible from senior colleagues too; many remember their MRCP exam vividly and are keen to assist you in gaining those four precious letters after your name.

The day before

Check that you have your examination paperwork in order with your examination number as well as where and what time you are needed – you don't want to get lost or be late. Also ensure that you have packed some identification (e.g. a passport) as you will need this to register on the day. Remember to take with you vital equipment you are familiar with using, particularly your stethoscope, although avoid weighing yourself down with cotton wool, pins, otoscope and so on. The necessary equipment will be provided for you. Punctuality is important and reduces stress, so we advise that you travel to your exam the day before, unless your exam centre is on your doorstep. Avoid last-minute revision and try to relax – you will certainly know enough by now. Spend the evening doing something other than medicine and get an early night!

On the day

Think carefully about your attire – first impressions count both with the examiners and more importantly with the patients. Broadly speaking, exam dress policy is similar to that required of NHS employees. You should look smart and professional, but above all wear something that is comfortable. Shirts should be open collar (not low cut) and short sleeved to enable bare-below-the-elbow and effective hand sanitation. Remove watches/jewellery (wedding bands are permitted) and dangling necklaces/chains that could be distracting or hit the patient. Facial piercings other than ear studs are not recommended.

Examination

You will have 16 mark sheets – two for each encounter. There will be a short problem-orientated clinical question with an instruction prior to starting the station encounter, for example 'This man has been inadvertently dropping things – please assess his upper limbs neurologically' or 'This woman has been complaining of breathlessness – please assess her cardiovascular system'. Use the preparatory time before each case wisely and remember to answer the question when presenting your findings.

When you enter the station encounter, hand the mark sheets to the examiners and remember to **HIT** it off with the examiners and the patient:

- Hand sanitization (if available).
- Introduce yourself to the patient and ask permission to examine them.
- Take a step back once the patient is appropriately uncovered/positioned and spend 20 seconds observing them closely. This is roughly the time it takes for hand sanitizer to dry. It can feel an extraordinarily long period of time when under exam conditions but it is time well spent. As soon as you start touching the patient, your focus becomes blinkered and you will miss vital peripheral clues to the case.

Remembering to HIT it off will help settle your nerves and then you'll be underway. The rest will follow fluently if you are well practised.

Rather like when looking in the rear-view mirror in a driving test, be sure to convey to your examiner what you are doing. Try not to move the patient excessively and repeatedly; your examiner will be expecting to see you do things in an efficient and familiar order and doing so looks systematic, practised and fluent. However, if you do forget to do something halfway through the examination, or you have to go back to check a physical finding, that's fine. It's more important to be comprehensive and sure of the clinical findings than just to try to be 'slick'.

Spend the last few moments of your examination time working out what is going on, what the diagnosis is and what you are going to say to the examiner. There's still time to check again. Most examinations can be completed by standing up and saying to the examiners a phrase like 'To complete my examination I would like to check…' and then listing a few things you may have omitted and/or are important to the case, such as blood pressure, urine dipstick and so on.

Presentation

Eye contact and a direct, unambiguous presentation of the case convey confidence and reassure examiners that you are on top of things. Avoid the phrases 'I'm not sure if it is…' and 'I think it is…' Be definitive and avoid sitting on the fence, but above all be honest. Don't make up clinical signs to fit a specific diagnosis (some cases may be normal to assess your ability to detect the absence of signs). Try not to present clinical signs that are inconsistent with the diagnosis or differential diagnosis.

There are two ways to present the case:

- State the diagnosis and support this with key positive and negative clinical findings – if (and only if) you are confident you have secured the correct diagnosis.
- State the relevant positive and negative clinical signs (it's often easier to do this in the order you elicited them) and then give the differential diagnosis that is consistent with these – particularly if you are unsure of the diagnosis.

Where possible, you should comment on the disease severity or disease activity. Consider complications of the diagnosis and mention if these are present or not. Know when to stop talking. Brevity can be an asset: it avoids you making mistakes and digging a hole for yourself! Wait for the examiners to ask a question and do not be pre-emptive – the examiners may follow you down the rabbit hole and possibly expose a gap in your knowledge.

Examiners

Prior to you examining the patient the examiners will have individually 'calibrated the case' to assess its difficulty and ensure that the clinical signs are present. This maintains the fairness and robustness of the exam and makes sure consistency exists in exam centre marking. There will be two examiners for every carousel station and usually one will lead the discussion with you. Both will have the mark sheets that you gave them at the start of the encounter and will mark you independently without collaboration. Contrary to popular belief, they both want you to pass. They are there because they are Fellows of the College in good standing and support the training and progression of the talented physicians of the future.

Mistakes happen

If you do make a mistake and realize it, don't be afraid to correct yourself. To err is human and the examiners may overlook a minor faux pas or mis-speak if the rest of the case has gone well. It's not uncommon to think that you have failed a case halfway round the carousel and that your chances of passing PACES have been dealt a fatal blow. We are often our own harshest critics, so don't write yourself off. Frequently, all is not lost. Don't let your performance dip on the next cases because you are still reeling from the last. Put any mistakes behind you and *keep calm and carry on*!

Respiratory

Clinical mark sheet

Clinical skill	Satisfactory	Unsatisfactory
Physical examination	Correct, thorough, fluent, systematic, professional	Incorrect technique, omits, unsystematic, hesitant
Identifying physical signs	Identifies correct signs Does not find signs that are not present	Misses important signs Finds signs that are not present
Differential diagnosis	Constructs sensible differential diagnosis	Poor differential, fails to consider the correct diagnosis
Clinical judgement	Sensible and appropriate management plan	Inappropriate management Unfamiliar with management
Maintaining patient welfare	Respectful, sensitive Ensures comfort, safety and dignity	Causes physical or emotional discomfort Jeopardizes patient safety

Cases for PACES, Fourth Edition. Stephen Hoole, Andrew Fry and Rachel Davies.
© 2025 John Wiley & Sons Ltd. Published 2025 by John Wiley & Sons Ltd.

Respiratory exam – general advice

- You should be trying to get as many clues to the diagnosis as possible before you lay a hand on the patient
- The patient will already have their chest exposed and will usually be sitting comfortably at 45 degrees
- Introduce yourself and ensure that the patient appears comfortable
- Take a step back to the end of the bed and spend 20 seconds looking at the patient and the area surrounding their bed. Use the following prompts to run through a list in your head to ensure that you are actively looking for information rather than just aimlessly staring
- What clues are you expecting to see from the end of the bed in the respiratory exam?
  - General body habitus – cachexia, Cushingoid features, paper-thin skin associated with steroid use, short stature secondary to respiratory illness starting in childhood (cystic fibrosis; bronchiectasis)
  - Sputum pot – look to see the colour; pistachio-coloured sputum often a sign of pseudomonas infection; pink – pulmonary haemorrhage
  - Inhalers – make sure you are familiar with new colours of these, particularly combination inhalers
  - Supplemental oxygen – watch for the presence of portable concentrators as opposed to cylinders that are now rarely used; may be in a 'rucksack' that is often navy in colour
  - Saddle-shaped nose – pulmonary vasculitis
  - Face – ptosis associated with Pancoast tumour
  - Tunnelled lines (upper chest) for delivery of medication in pulmonary hypertension patients or a portacath in a patient with cystic fibrosis
- At the end of the bed take a good look at the shape of the chest wall:
  - Are both sides moving together? Is one expanding further than the other? If one side is expanding less than the other then there might have been previous surgery on that side
  - Look at the shape of the chest – is there any deformity? Is it hyperexpanded?
  - Are there any scars on the anterior chest wall? Transplant scars, small scars in the xiphisternum suggestive of surgical chest drains during transplant or pulmonary endarterectomy (see pulmonary hypertension section)
  - Listen for a cough – dry may point towards pulmonary fibrosis, whereas a cough suggestive of the presence of sputum (more gurgling) might point to bronchiectasis or infection. This is a weak sign as well-treated patients with bronchiectasis may not currently produce sputum
  - Note the quality of the patient's voice. Enlarged pulmonary arteries stretch the recurrent laryngeal nerve leading to a hoarse voice and previous chest surgery may lead to damage to this nerve
- Ask the patient to hold their hands up in front of them:
  - Tremor – short-acting beta-agonist use if fine
  - Rheumatoid hands or those of scleroderma (PH)
  - Tar-stained fingers (smoker)
  - Nail signs – clubbing, rheumatoid nail changes
  - Get them to cock their wrists – asterixis ('CO_2 retention flap'); press gently back with your palm against their fingers and feel it if you're not sure
  - Wrist – take the pulse; CO_2 retention gives you a bounding pulse
- As you move up the arm, always state that you would like to measure the blood pressure at this point
- Examine the face, looking for:
  - Conjunctival pallor (pull down one eyelid with your little finger)
  - Signs of other systemic disease with respiratory pathology – scleroderma (beaked nose, small mouth with peri-oral furrowing), hereditary haemorrhagic telangiectasia (facial/oral telangiectasia)

- ○ Central cyanosis – lips and tongue
- ○ Facial palsy of a Pancoast tumour if not already spotted
- Briefly look for a significantly raised JVP while moving to examine the neck
- Examine for cervical lymphadenopathy
- Take a good look at the anterior and lateral chest wall for scars and also tattoo of radiotherapy. Also examine for well-healed mastectomy scars, as the patient may have had historical, poorly focused radiotherapy that caused localised damage to the lung resulting in fibrosis. If the patient seems comfortable you might wish to look at the posterior aspect of the thorax for surgical scars at this point. If they seem very breathless remember to do this when you examine the posterior aspect of the chest
- Examine for the trachea – place your index finger on the medial end of the right clavicle and your ring finger on the medial end of the left clavicle. Slowly move your middle finger up towards the sternal notch. You should find the trachea. If it is deviated, move your middle finger until it touches the trachea lightly. At this point your middle finger will be acting as a pointer to indicate which direction the trachea is deviated towards. Use the patient's right and left to describe the direction of deviation, i.e. towards the patient's right or left thorax
- Examine for chest expansion:
  - ○ Upper chest – place both hands flat on the apices of the lung; the expansion is a vertical movement. Use your own proprioception as well as watching to detect a difference in hand movement
  - ○ Mid-thoracic expansion is a lateral movement – ask the patient to take a deep breath in. Start by putting the edge of your index fingers on the chest with the rest of your hand perpendicular to the chest wall. Bring your thumbs towards the centre of the chest and ask the patient to take a deep breath out and then in again
  - ○ Examine the posterior chest expansion just once when you have finished examining the whole of the anterior chest. Use the mid-thoracic technique
- Then briefly examine the following anterior aspects of the chest before focusing on the posterior aspects, to avoid moving the patient too frequently:
  - ○ Detect the percussion note – in the upper, middle and lower zones. Look for a resonant (healthy lung), dull (consolidation) or stony dull (effusion) note. Loss of a dull percussion note over the heart may be a sign of emphysema
  - ○ Auscultate the anterior aspect in the upper and mid thorax and the posterior chest wall in six places. Move your stethoscope initially horizontally for the first two locations and then vertically down one in a zigzag pattern, which enables you to compare not only left to right but also vertical zones
- Move down to the legs to examine for peripheral oedema. Use these additional few moments to prepare in your head what you are going to say to the examiners as to your findings
- Turn round to face the examiners and state that you would also like to do some of the following:
  - ○ Measure the oxygen saturations
  - ○ Look in the sputum pot if you haven't already done this
  - ○ Perform a peak flow measurement if you feel the patient may have airways disease or a lung transplant

Pulmonary fibrosis
Examine this patient's respiratory system, she has been complaining of progressive shortness of breath.

Clinical signs
- Clubbing, central cyanosis and tachypnoea
- Fine end-inspiratory crackles (like Velcro® that do not change with coughing)
- Signs of associated autoimmune diseases, e.g. rheumatoid arthritis (hands), SLE and systemic sclerosis (face and hands)
- Signs of treatment, e.g. Cushingoid from steroids
- Discoloured skin (grey) – amiodarone
- Unless there are any associated features then describe your findings as pulmonary fibrosis, which is a clinical description pending further differentiation following investigations
- Beware single lung transplantation patient – unilateral fine crackles and contralateral thoracotomy scar with normal breath sounds

Discussion
INVESTIGATION
- **Bloods:** ESR, rheumatoid factor and ANA
- **CXR:** reticulonodular changes; loss of definition of either heart border; small lungs
- **ABG:** type I respiratory failure
- **Lung function tests:**
  - $FEV_1/FVC > 0.8$ (restrictive)
  - Low TLC (small lungs)
  - Reduced TL_{CO} and K_{CO}
- **Bronchoalveolar lavage:** main indication is to exclude any infection prior to immunosuppressants, plus if lymphocytes > neutrophils indicates a better response to steroids and a better prognosis (sarcoidosis)
- **High-resolution CT scan:** distribution helps with diagnosis; bi-basal subpleural honeycombing typical of UIP; widespread ground-glass shadowing more likely to be non-specific interstitial pneumonia often associated with autoimmune disease; if apical in distribution then think of sarcoidosis, ABPA, old TB, hypersensitivity pneumonitis, Langerhans cell histiocytosis. However, radiology needs to be reviewed in the context of other clinical parameters such as autoimmune profile
- **Lung biopsy** (associated morbidity ~7%)

TREATMENT
- Immunosuppression if likely to be inflammatory, e.g. steroids; combination of steroids and azathioprine no longer used following results of PANTHER trial that showed increased morbidity on this combination
- If thought to be IPF then the patient needs to be referred to an NHSE-recognised ILD service for consideration of an antifibrotic agent, e.g. pirfenidone – for when FEV_1 50–80% predicted (NICE recommended)
- Single lung transplant

PROGNOSIS
- Very variable – depends on aetiology
- Highly cellular with ground-glass infiltrate – responds to immunosuppression: 80% 5-year survival
- Honeycombing on CT – no response to immunosuppression: 80% 5-year mortality
- Increased risk of bronchogenic carcinoma

CAUSES OF BASAL FIBROSIS
- UIP
- Asbestosis
- Connective tissue diseases
- Aspiration – often asymmetrical crackles; R > L (right main bronchus is shorter, wider and straighter: foreign bodies more likely to enter)

Bronchiectasis

This 60-year-old woman presents to your clinic with a persistent cough. Please examine her and discuss your findings.

Clinical signs
- **General:** Cachexia and tachypnoea
- **Hands:** Clubbing
- **Chest:** Mixed-character crackles that alter with coughing. Occasional squeaks and wheeze. Sputum +++ (look in the pot!)
- **Cor pulmonale:** SOA, raised JVP, RV heave, loud P_2
- **Yellow nail syndrome:** yellow nails and lymphoedema

Discussion
INVESTIGATION
- Sputum culture and cytology
- **CXR:** tramlines and ring shadows
- **High-resolution CT thorax:** 'signet ring' sign (thickened, dilated bronchi larger than the adjacent vascular bundle)

FOR A SPECIFIC CAUSE
- Immunoglobulins: hypogammaglobulinaemia (especially IgG_2 and IgA)
- *Aspergillus* RAST or skin prick testing: ABPA (upper lobe)
- Rheumatoid serology
- Saccharine ciliary motility test (nares to taste buds in 30 minutes): Kartagener's
- Genetic screening: cystic fibrosis
- History of IBD: particularly post total pancolectomy in UC

CAUSES OF BRONCHIECTASIS
- **Congenital:** Kartagener's and cystic fibrosis
- **Childhood infection:** measles and TB
- **Immune *overactivity*:** ABPA; IBD associated
- **Immune *underactivity*:** hypogammaglobulinaemia; CVID
- **Aspiration:** chronic alcoholics; post stroke with swallowing problems and GORD; localized to right lower lobe

TREATMENT
- Physiotherapy – active cycle breathing
- Prompt antibiotic therapy for exacerbations
- Long-term treatment with low-dose azithromycin three times per week
- Bronchodilators/inhaled corticosteroids if there is any airflow obstruction
- Surgery is occasionally used for localized disease

COMPLICATIONS OF BRONCHIECTASIS
- Cor pulmonale
- (Secondary) amyloidosis (dip urine for protein)
- Massive haemoptysis (mycotic aneurysm)

Old tuberculosis

Please examine this man's respiratory system.

Clinical signs
- Chest deformity and absent ribs; thoracoplasty scar
- Tracheal deviation towards the side of the fibrosis (traction)
- Reduced expansion
- Dull percussion but present tactile vocal fremitus
- Crackles and bronchial breathing

Discussion

HISTORICAL TECHNIQUES
- Plombage: insertion of polystyrene balls into the thoracic cavity
- Phrenic nerve crush: diaphragm paralysis
- Thoracoplasty: rib removal; lung not resected
- Apical lobectomy
- Recurrent medical pneumothoraces
- Streptomycin was introduced in the 1950s and was the first drug shown to be beneficial for TB in a randomized controlled trial

SERIOUS SIDE EFFECTS OF TB DRUGS
- **Isoniazid:** peripheral neuropathy (Rx pyridoxine) and hepatitis
- **Rifampicin:** hepatitis and increased contraceptive pill metabolism
- **Ethambutol:** retrobulbar neuritis and hepatitis
- **Pyrazinamide:** hepatitis

Prior to treating TB, check baseline liver function tests and visual acuity. Tell the patient the following:

- Look at the whites of your eyes every morning. If yellow, stop the tablets and ring the TB nurse that morning
- Notice colours – if red becomes less bright than you expect, ring the TB nurse that day
- You may develop tingling in your toes – continue with the tablets but tell the doctor at your next clinic visit
- Your secretions will turn orange/red because of a dye in one of the tablets. If you wear contact lenses they will become permanently stained and should not be worn
- If you are on the OCP, it may fail. Use barrier contraception

CAUSES OF APICAL FIBROSIS: 'TRASH'
- **T**B
- **R**adiation
- **A**nkylosing spondylitis/**A**BPA
- **S**arcoidosis
- **H**istoplasmosis/**H**istiocytosis X/**H**ypersensitivity pneumonitis)

Surgical respiratory cases

Please examine this man who initially presented to doctors with a cough and weight loss.

Lobectomy

- Reduced expansion and chest wall deformity
- Thoracotomy scar: same for either upper or lower lobe
- Trachea is central
- Lower lobectomy: dull percussion note over lower zone with absent breath sounds
- Upper lobectomy: may have normal examination or may have a hyper-resonant percussion note over upper zone with a dull percussion note at base where the hemidiaphragm is elevated slightly

- **CXR:** may be no overt abnormality apparent other than slight raised hemidiaphragm; remember that the right hemidiaphragm should be higher than the left in health
- **CT chest:** loss of a lobe with associated truncation of bronchus or pulmonary vessels

Pneumonectomy

- Thoracotomy scar (indistinguishable from thoracotomy scar performed for a lobectomy)
- Reduced expansion on the side of the pneumonectomy
- Trachea deviated towards the side of the pneumonectomy
- Dull percussion note throughout the hemithorax
- Absent tactile vocal fremitus beneath the thoracotomy scar
- Bronchial breathing in the upper zone with reduced breath sound throughout remainder of hemithorax (bronchial breathing is due to transmitted sound from major airways)

- CXR: complete white-out on side of pneumonectomy
- Pneumonectomy space fills with gelatinous material within a few weeks of the operation

Single lung transplant

- **Clinical signs:** thoracotomy scar; normal exam on side of scar; may have clinical signs on opposite hemithorax
- **Indications for 'dry lung' conditions:** COPD; pulmonary fibrosis

Double lung transplant

- **Clinical signs:** clamshell incision – from the one axilla along the line of the lower ribs up to the xiphisternum to the other axilla
- **Indications for 'wet lung' conditions:** CF, bronchiectasis or pulmonary hypertension

Chronic obstructive airways disease
Please examine this patient's chest; he has a chronic chest condition.

Clinical signs
- Inspection: nebulizer/inhalers/sputum pot, dyspnoea, central cyanosis and pursed lips
- CO_2 retention flap, bounding pulse and tar-stained fingers
- Hyper-expanded
- Percussion note resonant with loss of cardiac dullness
- Expiratory polyphonic wheeze (crackles if consolidation too) and reduced breath sounds at apices
- Cor pulmonale: raised JVP, ankle oedema, RV heave; loud P_2 with pansystolic murmur of tricuspid regurgitation
- COPD does not cause clubbing, therefore if present consider bronchial carcinoma or bronchiectasis

Discussion
- Spectrum of disease with airway obstruction (with or without sputum production); can be low FEV_1 at one end and emphysema with low O_2 sats and TL_{CO} but normal spirometry at the other
- Degree of overlap with chronic asthma, although in COPD there is less reversibility (<15% change in FEV_1 post bronchodilators)

CAUSES
- **Environmental:** smoking and industrial dust exposure (apical disease)
- **Genetic:** α_1-antitrypsin deficiency (predominantly basal disease)

INVESTIGATIONS
- **CXR:** hyper-expanded and/or pneumothorax
- **ABG:** type II respiratory failure (low PaO_2, high $PaCO_2$)
- **Bloods:** high WCC (infection), low α_1-antitrypsin (younger patients/FH+), low albumin (severity)
- **Spirometry:** low FEV_1, FEV_1/FVC <0.7 (obstructive)
- **Gas transfer:** low TL_{CO}

TREATMENT
- **Medical** – depends on severity (GOLD classification):
  - Smoking cessation is the single most beneficial management strategy
  - Cessation clinics and nicotine replacement therapy
  - Long-term oxygen therapy (LTOT)
  - Pulmonary rehabilitation
  - Mild (FEV_1 >80%) – beta-agonists
  - Moderate (FEV_1 <60%) – tiotropium plus beta-agonists
  - Severe (FEV_1 <40%) or frequent exacerbations – as for moderate plus inhaled corticosteroids, although avoid if patient has ever had an episode of pneumonia (TORCH trial). Triple inhalers are now available, which improves adherence to therapy
  - Exercise
  - Nutrition (often malnourished)
  - Vaccinations – pneumococcal and influenza
- **Surgical** – careful patient selection is important:
  - Bullectomy (if bullae >1 L and compresses surrounding lung)
  - Endobronchial valve placement
  - Lung reduction surgery: only suitable for a few patients with heterogeneous distribution of emphysema
  - Single lung transplant

LONG-TERM OXYGEN THERAPY (LTOT)
- **Inclusion criteria:**
  - Non-smoker
  - PaO_2 <7.3 kPa on air
  - $PaCO_2$ that does not rise excessively on O_2
  - If evidence of cor pulmonale, PaO_2 <8 kPa
- 2–4 L/min via nasal prongs for at least 15 hours a day
- Improves average survival by 9 months

TREATMENT OF AN ACUTE EXACERBATION
- Controlled O_2 via Venturi mask monitored closely
- Bronchodilators
- Antibiotics
- Steroids 7 days

PROGNOSIS
- COPD patients with an acute exacerbation have 15% in-hospital mortality

DIFFERENTIAL OF A WHEEZY CHEST
- **Granulomatous polyarteritis** (previously Wegner's): saddle nose; obliterative bronchiolitis
- **Rheumatoid arthritis:** wheeze secondary to obliterative bronchiolitis
- **Post lung transplant:** obliterative bronchiolitis as part of chronic rejection spectrum

Pleural effusion

This patient has been breathless for 2 weeks. Examine his respiratory system to elucidate the cause.

Clinical signs

- Asymmetrically reduced expansion
- Trachea or mediastinum displaced away from the side of the effusion
- **Stony** dull percussion note
- Absent tactile vocal fremitus
- Reduced breath sounds
- Bronchial breathing above the effusion (aegophony)

SIGNS THAT MAY INDICATE THE CAUSE

- **Cancer:** clubbing; lymphadenopathy; mastectomy (breast cancer being a very common cause of pleural effusion)
- **Congestive cardiac failure:** raised JVP; peripheral oedema
- **Chronic liver disease:** leuconychia, spider naevi, gynaecomastia
- **Chronic renal failure:** arteriovenous fistula
- **Connective tissue disease:** rheumatoid hands; facial butterfly rash of SLE

CAUSES OF A DULL LUNG BASE

- **Consolidation:** bronchial breathing and crackles
- **Collapse:** tracheal deviation towards the side of collapse and reduced breath sounds
- **Previous lobectomy** = reduced lung volume
- **Pleural thickening:** signs are similar to a pleural effusion but with normal tactile vocal fremitus; may have three scars suggestive of previous VATS pleurodesis
- **Raised hemidiaphragm** ± hepatomegaly

Discussion

CAUSES

Transudate (protein <30 g/L)	Exudate (protein >30 g/L)
Congestive cardiac failure	Neoplasm: 1° or 2°
Chronic renal failure	Infection
Chronic liver failure	Infarction
	Inflammation: RA and SLE

INVESTIGATIONS

- **CXR:** white-out with blunting and loss of costophrenic angle and (if large) loss of heart border with a meniscus-shaped contour on erect PA radiograph. No associated mediastinal shift suggests lung collapse and possible bronchial obstruction
- CT chest
- Pleural tap, drain, biopsy (CT-guided or VATS) may be diagnostic
- Bronchoscopy

Pleural aspiration (exudate)

- **Protein:** effusion albumin/plasma albumin >0.5 (Light's criteria)
- **LDH:** effusion LDH/plasma LDH >0.6
- **Empyema:** exudate with low glucose and pH <7.2 is suggestive

Empyema

- Collection of pus within the pleural space
- Most frequent organisms anaerobes, staphylococci and Gram-negative organisms
- Associated with bronchial obstruction, e.g. carcinoma, with recurrent aspiration; poor dentition; alcohol dependence

Mesothelioma

- Tumour affecting the pleura and occasionally pericardium or peritoneum
- Associated with asbestos exposure in 80% of cases, pleural plaques on CXR and effusion

TREATMENT

- Pleural drainage
- If recurrent consider pleurodesis, pleuro-peritoneal 'window', VATS pleurectomy/ decortication
- **Empyema:** IV antibiotics and intrapleural DNase plus tPA (MIST2 trial)
- **Mesothelioma:** surgery and chemotherapy, although treatment response is often poor

Lung cancer
Please examine this patient who has had a three-month history of chronic cough, malaise and weight loss.

Clinical signs
- Cachectic
- Clubbing and tar-stained fingers
- Lymphadenopathy: cervical and axillary
- Tracheal deviation: towards (collapse) or away (effusion) from the lesion
- Reduced expansion
- Percussion note dull (collapse/consolidation) or stony dull (effusion)
- Absent tactile vocal fremitus (effusion); increased vocal resonance (collapse/consolidation)
- Auscultation:
  - Crackles and bronchial breathing (consolidation/collapse)
  - Reduced breath sounds; absent tactile fremitus (effusion)
- **Hepatomegaly or bony tenderness:** metastasis
- **Treatment:**
  - Lobectomy scar
  - Radiotherapy: square burn and tattoo
- Complications:
  - **Superior vena cava obstruction:** suffused and oedematous face and upper limbs, dilated superficial chest veins and stridor
  - **Recurrent laryngeal nerve palsy:** hoarse with a 'bovine' cough
  - **Horner's sign and wasted small muscles of the hand (T1):** Pancoast's tumour
  - **Endocrine:** gynaecomastia (ectopic βHCG)
  - **Neurological:** Lambert–Eaton myasthenia syndrome, peripheral neuropathy, proximal myopathy and paraneoplastic cerebellar degeneration
  - **Dermatological:** dermatomyositis (heliotrope rash on eyelids and purple papules on knuckles (Gottron's papules associated with a raised CK) and acanthosis nigricans

Discussion
TYPES
- Squamous 35%, small (oat) 24%, adeno 21%, large 19% and alveolar 1%

MANAGEMENT
1. Diagnosis of a mass:
   - **CXR:** collapse, mass and hilar lymphadenopathy
   - **Volume acquisition CT thorax** (so small tumours are not lost between slices) with contrast
2. Determine cell type:
   - **Induced sputum cytology**
   - **Biopsy** by **bronchoscopy** (central lesion and collapse) or **percutaneous needle** CT guided (peripheral lesion; FEV_1 >1 L)
3. Stage – **CT/bronchoscopy/endobronchial ultrasound-guided biopsy/ mediastinoscopy/thoracoscopy/PET:**
   - **Non-small cell carcinoma (NSCLC):** TNM staging to assess operability
   - **Small cell carcinoma (SCLC):** previously divided into limited or extensive disease, now has its own TNM staging classification
4. Lung function tests for operability assessment:
   - Pneumonectomy contraindicated if FEV_1 <1.2 L
5. Complications of the tumour:
   - Metastasis: ↑ LFTs, ↑ Ca^{++}, ↓ Hb
   - NSCLC: ↑ PTHrP → ↑ Ca^{++}
   - SCLC: ↑ ACTH, SIADH → ↓ Na^+

TREATMENT

- **NSCLC:**
  - **Surgery:** lobectomy or pneumonectomy
  - **Radiotherapy:** single fractionation (weekly) versus hyper-fractionation (daily for 10 days)
  - **Chemotherapy:** benefit unknown; eGFR positive – erlotinib
- **SCLC:**
  - **Chemotherapy:** benefit with six courses
- A multidisciplinary approach is important

PALLIATIVE CARE

- Dexamethasone and radiotherapy for brain metastasis
- SVCO: dexamethasone plus radiotherapy or intravascular stent
- Radiotherapy for haemoptysis, bone pain and cough
- Chemical pleurodesis for effusion – talc; tetracycline no longer used
- Opiates for cough and pain

PROGNOSIS

- Surveillance, Epidemiology and End Results (SEER) stage predicts the 5-year survival rate for SCLC:
  - Localised: 27%
  - Regional: 16%
  - Distant: 3%
  - All stages combined: 6%
- The 5-year survival for NSCLC of all stages combined is 24%

Cystic fibrosis

Please examine this young man's chest and comment on what you find.

Clinical signs

- Inspection: small stature, **clubbed**, tachypnoeic, sputum pot (purulent++)
- Hyperinflated with reduced chest expansion
- **Coarse crackles** and wheeze (bronchiectatic)
- **Portex reservoir** (portacath) under the skin or **Hickman line/scars** for long-term antibiotics plus PEG for malabsorption

Discussion

GENETICS

- Incidence of 1/2500 live births
- Autosomal recessive chromosome 7q
- Gene encodes CFTR (Cl⁻ channel)
- Commonest and most severe mutation is deletion ΔF508-CFTR (70%)

PATHOPHYSIOLOGY

Secretions are thickened and block the lumens of various structures:

- Bronchioles → bronchiectasis
- Pancreatic ducts → loss of exocrine and endocrine function
- Gut → distal intestinal obstruction syndrome (DIOS) in adults
- Seminal vesicles → male infertility
- Fallopian tubes – reduced female fertility

INVESTIGATIONS

- Screened at birth: low immunoreactive trypsin (heel prick)
- Sweat test: Na⁺ >60 mmol/L (false positive in hypothyroidism and Addison's)
- Genetic screening

TREATMENT

- **Physiotherapy:** postural drainage and active cycle breathing techniques
- Prompt antibiotics for intercurrent infections
- Pancrease® and fat-soluble vitamin supplements
- Mucolytics (DNase)
- Immunizations
- CFTR modulators – for adults with suitable CFTR mutations (~90% of CF patients)
  - Improve production and function of the receptor
  - Importantly improve intracellular trafficking of receptor to the cell membrane
  - In homozygous Δ508 patients triple therapy with Trikafta® showed significant improvement in FEV_1 % and QoL with a 60% reduction in infective exacerbations in 4 weeks
- Double lung transplant (50% survival at 5 years)
- Gene therapy is under development

PROGNOSIS

- Median survival is 40 years but is rising.
- Poor prognosis if becomes infected with *Burkholderia cepacia*.

Pneumonia

This patient has been acutely unwell for 3 days, with shortness of breath and a productive cough. Please examine his chest.

Clinical signs

- Tachypnoea, O_2 mask, sputum pot (rusty sputum associated with pneumococcus)
- Reduced expansion
- Dull percussion note
- Focal coarse crackles, increased vocal resonance and bronchial breathing
- Ask for the temperature chart
- If dull percussion note with absent tactile vocal fremitus, think parapneumonic effusion/empyema

Discussion

INVESTIGATION

- **CXR:** consolidation (air bronchogram), abscess and effusion
- **Bloods:** WCC, CRP, urea, atypical serology (on admission and at day 10) and immunoglobulins
- **Blood** (25% positive) and **sputum cultures**
- **Urine:**
  - ○ *Legionella* antigen (in severe cases)
  - ○ Pneumococcal antigen
  - ○ Haemoglobinuria (*Mycoplasma* causes cold agglutinins → haemolysis)

COMMUNITY-ACQUIRED PNEUMONIA (CAP)

- Common organisms:
  - ○ ***Streptococcus pneumoniae*** 50%
  - ○ ***Mycoplasma pneumoniae*** 6%
  - ○ *Haemophilus influenzae* (especially if COPD)
  - ○ *Chlamydia pneumoniae*
- Antibiotics:
  - ○ First line: penicillin *or* cephalosporin + macrolide

SPECIAL CONSIDERATIONS

- **Immunosuppressed:**
  - ○ Fungal Rx: amphotericin
  - ○ Multi-resistant mycobacteria
  - ○ *Pneumocystis carinii*: Rx co-trimoxazole/pentamidine
  - ○ CMV: Rx ganciclovir
- **Aspiration** (commonly posterior segment of right lower lobe):
  - ○ Anaerobes: Rx + metronidazole
- **Post influenza:**
  - ○ *Staph. aureus*: Rx + flucloxacillin

SEVERITY SCORE FOR PNEUMONIA: CURB-65 (2/5 IS SEVERE)

- **C**onfusion
- **U**rea >7
- **R**espiratory rate >30
- **B**P systolic <90 mm Hg or diastolic <60 mm Hg
- **A**ge >65

Severe CAP should receive high-dose IV antibiotics initially plus level 2 care (HDU/ITU)

- Pneumovax® II to high-risk groups, e.g. chronic disease (especially nephrotic and asplenic patients) and the elderly

COMPLICATIONS
- Lung abscess (*Staph. aureus*, *Klebsiella*, anaerobes)
- Para-pneumonic effusion/empyema
- Haemoptysis
- Septic shock and multi-organ failure

Pulmonary hypertension

This 35-year-old woman presents to your clinic with shortness of breath and syncope. Please examine her and discuss your findings.

Clinical signs

- **General:** often looks very healthy. May have a central tunnelled catheter for administration of continuous IV epoprostenol or a hand-held, battery-operated nebulizer next to the bed for iloprost. Peripheral oedema. Mid-line thoracotomy scar indicates pulmonary endarterectomy surgery
- **Hands:** clubbing if associated with congenital heart disease; features of scleroderma
- **JVP:** raised – may have systemic V waves associated with tricuspid regurgitation; if euvolaemic and well treated may not be raised
- **Chest:** lungs will be clear. Listen for the heart sounds at the right sternal edge for the murmur of tricuspid regurgitation
- **Ask the examiner:** oxygen saturations – preferably after walking up and down the corridor

Discussion

INVESTIGATION

- Echocardiography – looking for right ventricular size and function, peak tricuspid regurgitant velocity to estimate systolic pulmonary pressure
- If intermediate to high probability of pulmonary hypertension on echo, identify an underlying cause to guide treatment
- **Blood tests:** autoimmune screen (scleroderma and SLE); thyroid function (hyperthyroidism); liver function (porto-pulmonary PH); HIV
- **Imaging:** CTPA (looking for proximal chronic thrombi but also parenchymal lung disease); VQ (distal chronic thrombi); US abdomen (portal hypertension)
- **Physiology:** lung function (underlying lung disease – ILD or COPD)
- **Right heart catheterization:** confirmation of raised pulmonary pressures plus estimation of left atrial pressure (wedge pressure) to guide left heart function

CAUSES

WHO Clinical Classification – diseases grouped according to pathophysiology but also response to treatment

- **Group 1 – pulmonary arterial hypertension (PAH):** idiopathic; heritable (*BMPR2* mutations); drugs and toxins (amphetamines; TKI desatinib); connective tissue disease; congenital heart disease; portal hypertension; HIV; schistosomiasis
- **Group 2 – left heart disease:** systolic or diastolic dysfunction or valvular disease
- **Group 3 – lung disease:** COPD; ILD; obesity hypoventilation; sarcoidosis
- **Group 4** – chronic thromboembolic disease
- **Group 5 – miscellaneous:** including long-term haemodialysis and thyrotoxicosis

TREATMENT

- **Group 1 – PAH:** pulmonary vasodilators: phosphodiesterase 5 inhibitors (sildenafil, tadalafil); endothelin receptor antagonists (macitentan, ambrisentan); prostacyclin analogues (epoprostenol administered by continuous intravenous infusion; iloprost – nebulized; oral selexipag); double lung transplant
- **Group 4** – chronic thromboembolic pulmonary hypertension: lifelong anticoagulation; if proximal, pulmonary endarterectomy surgery; if distal, balloon pulmonary angioplasty and soluble guanylate cyclase stimulator (riociguat)
- **Groups 2, 3 and most of 5** – targeted pulmonary hypertension treatment is contraindicated; treat the underlying cause

COMPLICATIONS

- Death from right heart failure
- Atrial arrhythmias
- Dilatation of the proximal pulmonary artery – stretching of the recurrent laryngeal nerve (hoarse voice); external compression of the left anterior descending artery (angina-like chest pain and ventricular arrhythmias); external compression of the right middle lobe bronchus (localized bronchiectasis)

Cardiology

Clinical mark sheet

Clinical skill	Satisfactory	Unsatisfactory
Physical examination	Correct, thorough, fluent, systematic, professional	Incorrect technique, omits, unsystematic, hesitant
Identifying physical signs	Identifies correct signs Does not find signs that are not present	Misses important signs Finds signs that are not present
Differential diagnosis	Constructs sensible differential diagnosis	Poor differential, fails to consider the correct diagnosis
Clinical judgement	Sensible and appropriate management plan	Inappropriate management Unfamiliar with management
Maintaining patient welfare	Respectful, sensitive Ensures comfort, safety and dignity	Causes physical or emotional discomfort Jeopardizes patient safety

Cases for PACES, Fourth Edition. Stephen Hoole, Andrew Fry and Rachel Davies.
© 2025 John Wiley & Sons Ltd. Published 2025 by John Wiley & Sons Ltd.

Cardiology exam – general advice

- Expose the patient's chest. A gown that opens at the front may be provided for female patients but remember that this may hide valuable signs. Position the patient head up at 45 degrees
- What clues are you expecting to see (hear) from the end of the bed?
  - Scars from surgery or devices, abdominal bruising from LMWH
  - Mechanical heart valve clicks
  - GTN spray by the side of the bed
- Ask the patient to hold their hands up in front of them:
  - Nail signs: splinter haemorrhages, clubbing
  - Osler's nodes, Janeway lesions
  - Wrist: radial pulse, rate and rhythm; radio-femoral delay
- As you move up the arm:
  - Collapsing pulse: flat of the hand on the forearm flexor muscle bellies (ask about shoulder pain before elevating). A collapsing pulse is easily palpable striking all the fingers of the palmar surface of the examining hand
  - Ask for the blood pressure at this point – you may forget later
- Examine the face, looking for:
  - Eyes: corneal arcus, conjunctival pallor (pull down one eyelid with your little finger), xanthelasma
  - Cheeks: malar flush
  - Mouth: dentition, central cyanosis
- Neck:
  - Carotid pulse character, e.g. slow rising and bruit
  - JVP – is it raised? You will not be expected to diagnose constriction from the JVP so don't linger too long!
    - Support the patient's head relaxed on the pillow turned away from you and look across the neck obliquely for the biphasic waveform at the meniscus. Avoid pressing on the external jugular to fill it – it looks clumsy. If you can't see it, say so. Be prepared to state what you would do next to see it
    - High JVP: sit the patient at 90 degrees and/or deep inspiration – the meniscus will drop
    - Low JVP: lie the patient flatter or demonstrate the hepatojugular reflux – compressing the RUQ for 10 seconds – normally temporarily rises for a couple of beats (sustained rise suggests right heart failure)
- Precordium:
  - Check again for scars and devices
  - Feel for the apex beat and count the rib spaces. Ask yourself what the character is – heaving or thrusting, double impulse or tapping?
  - With the tips of your fingers feel for thrills in the aortic and pulmonary areas – palpable high-velocity jets?
  - With the heel of your right hand and a locked straight elbow, feel for a heave
  - Auscultation:
    - Heart sounds: loud or soft, mechanical, fixed split? Murmurs – systolic or diastolic? You may time the murmur with the upstroke of the carotid pulse
    - Use the bell at the apex for low-pitched rumbles, e.g. MS and AR, and the diaphragm for higher-pitched murmurs, e.g. MR and AS
    - Is there any radiation to axilla or carotids and can you make the murmur louder with inspiration or expiration or by positioning the patient in left lateral, sitting the patient forward, standing from squatting?
    - Use this time to put the auscultatory signs together with the peripheral findings to make a coherent diagnosis. How severe is the cardiac lesion? What is the cause and what are the effects?
    - Do you need to go back and check a peripheral sign?

- While the patient is sat forward look/palpate for sacral oedema and examine the chest
- Legs:
  - Scars from graft harvest site or varicose veins with venous eczema
  - Peripheral oedema: compress the medial malleoli gently while facing the patient at the end of the bed and check the patient's face to make sure this is not causing discomfort. Is the oedema pitting? If it is, how high up the leg does the swelling go?
  - Peripheral pulses
- Turn around to face the examiners and state that you would also like to do some of the following to complete your examination:
  - Perform fundoscopy – Roth spots (rarely), AV nipping, etc.
  - Check the blood pressure (if you forgot earlier)
  - Perform urinalysis

Aortic stenosis

This patient presents with increasing dyspnoea. Examine his cardiovascular system to elucidate the cause.

Clinical signs

- Slow-rising, low-volume pulse
- Narrow pulse pressure, e.g. 110/80 mm Hg
- Apex beat is **s**ustained in **s**tenosis (**HP: h**eaving **p**ressure loaded)
- Thrill in aortic area (right sternal edge, second intercostal space)
- Auscultation:

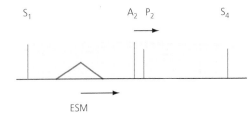

A loud, high-pitched, crescendo–decrescendo ejection systolic murmur (ESM), loudest in the aortic area during expiration and radiating to the carotids.

- **Severe** if soft and delayed A_2 due to immobile leaflets and prolonged LV emptying, delayed (not loud) ESM, fourth heart sound S_4 when in sinus rhythm
- **Complications:**
  - **Endocarditis:** splinters, Osler's nodes (finger pulp), Janeway lesions (palms), Roth spots (retina), temperature, splenomegaly and haematuria
  - **Left ventricular dysfunction:** dyspnoea, displaced apex and bi-basal crackles
  - **Pulmonary hypertension and right ventricular** failure are pre-terminal
  - **Conduction problems: acute**, endocarditis; **chronic**, calcified aortic valve node

Discussion

DIFFERENTIAL DIAGNOSIS OF ESM
- HOCM
- VSD
- Aortic sclerosis: normal pulse character and no radiation of murmur
- Aortic flow: high-output clinical states, e.g. pregnancy or anaemia

CAUSES OF AS
- Congenital: bicuspid (younger age)
- Acquired: **a**ge (senile degeneration and calcification); **s**treptococcal (rheumatic)

ASSOCIATIONS
- Coarctation and bicuspid aortic valve
- Angiodysplasia

SEVERITY

Symptom	50% mortality at
Angina	5 years
Syncope	3 years
Breathlessness	2 years

INVESTIGATIONS
- **ECG:** LVH on voltage criteria, conduction defect (prolonged PR interval)
- **CXR:** often normal; calcified valve
- **Echo:** mean gradient >40 mm Hg aortic (valve area <1.0 cm²) if severe, LV function
- **ETT:** symptoms, fall in BP
- **CT:** calcification (severity), annulus size, coronary and peripheral artery patency
- **Cardiac catheter:** invasive transvalvular gradient and coronary angiography (coronary artery disease often coexists with aortic stenosis)

MANAGEMENT
Asymptomatic:
- None specific, good dental health
- Regular review: symptoms and echo to assess gradient and LV function
- May be referred for intervention if LVEF <50% and low surgical risk

Symptomatic:
- **Surgical:**
  - Aortic valve replacement (sAVR) ± CABG
  - Operative mortality 3–5% depending on the patient's logistic EuroSCORE I or II: www.euroscore.org/calc.html
- **Percutaneous:**
  - Balloon aortic valvuloplasty (BAV)
  - Transcutaneous aortic valve implantation (TAVI)
    - Transfemoral (or trans-apical, -aortic, -subclavian, -carotid or -cavo-aortic)
    - In high surgical risk (log EuroSCORE >20%) or inoperable cases (number needed to treat to prevent death at 1 year = 5)
- Decision made at TAVI MDT by Heart Team:

Clinical Characteristics	Favours TAVI	Favours sAVR
Log EuroSCORE II ≥4% or I ≥10%	+	
Age ≥75	+	
Previous cardiac surgery	+	
Frailty	+	
Suspicious of endocarditis		+
Technical Aspects		
Unfavourable arterial access		+
Chest radiation	+	
Porcelain aorta	+	
Low coronary ostia		+
Large annulus (exceeds TAVI range)		+
Bicuspid or severe AR		+
Indication for other cardiac surgery		+

ESC Guideline 2017

Duke's criteria for infective endocarditis:

- Major:
  - Typical organism in two blood cultures
  - Echo: **abscess*, large vegetation*, dehiscence***
- **Minor:**
  - Pyrexia >38°C
  - Echo suggestive
  - Predisposed, e.g. prosthetic valve
  - **Embolic phenomena***
  - Vasculitic phenomena (ESR↑, CRP↑)
  - Atypical organism on blood culture
- * Plus **heart failure/refractory to antibiotics/heart block** – indicators for urgent surgery

Diagnose if the patient has 2 major, 1 major and 2 minor, or 5 minor criteria

Antibiotic prophylaxis is now limited to those with **prosthetic valves, previous endocarditis, cardiac transplants with valvopathy** and **certain types of congenital heart disease**

Aortic incompetence

This patient has been referred by his GP with 'a new murmur'. He is asymptomatic. Please examine his cardiovascular system and diagnose his problem.

Clinical signs
- Collapsing pulse (water-hammer pulse) reflecting a wide pulse pressure, e.g. 180/45 mm Hg
- Apex beat is hyperkinetic and displaced laterally (**TV: t**hrusting **v**olume-loaded)
- Thrill in the aortic area
- Auscultation:

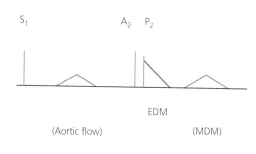

S_1 A_2 P_2

EDM

(Aortic flow)   (MDM)

A soft, high-pitched early diastolic murmur (EDM) loudest at the lower left sternal edge with the patient sat forward in expiration. There may be an aortic flow murmur and a low-pitched rumbling mid-diastolic murmur (MDM) (Austin–Flint) at the apex due to regurgitant flow impeding mitral opening.

- **Severe if:** EDM short (high LVEDP results in earlier pressure equalization) or silent ('free flow'), collapsing pulse, third heart sound (S_3) and pulmonary oedema
- **Eponymous signs:**
  - Corrigan's: visible vigorous neck pulsation
  - Quincke's: nail bed capillary pulsation
  - De Musset's: head nodding
  - Duroziez's: diastolic murmur proximal to femoral artery compression
  - Traube's: 'pistol shot' sound over the femoral arteries

Discussion
CAUSES
- Congenital: bicuspid aortic valve; peri-membranous VSD
- Acquired:

	Acute	Chronic
Valve leaflet	Endocarditis	Rheumatic fever
		Drugs: pergolide, slimming agents
Aortic root	Dissection (type A)	Dilatation: Marfan's and hypertension
	Trauma	Aortitis: syphilis, ankylosing spondylitis and vasculitis

OTHER CAUSES OF A COLLAPSING PULSE
- Pregnancy
- Patent ductus arteriosus
- Paget's disease
- Anaemia
- Thyrotoxicosis

INVESTIGATION
- **ECG:** lateral T-wave inversion
- **CXR:** cardiomegaly, widened mediastinum and pulmonary oedema
- **CT:** size of aortic root, dissection, coronary patency
- **TTE/TOE:** LVEF size, aortic root size/dissection, vegetation, jet width
- **Cardiac catheter:** coronary patency (usually pre-op)

MANAGEMENT
- Medical:
  - ACE inhibitors and ARBs (reducing afterload)
  - Regular review of symptoms and echo
- **Severity (on echo):**
  - LVEF (≤50%), LV size (ESD ≥50 mm and/or EDD ≥65 mm) and degree of AR (≥65% LVOT width)
- **Surgery – acute:**
  - Dissection
  - Aortic root abscess/endocarditis (homograft preferably)
- **Surgery – chronic:**
  Replace the aortic valve when:
  - **Symptomatic:** dyspnoea and reduced exercise tolerance (NYHA >II) **and/or**
  - **The following criteria are met:**
    1. Wide pulse pressure >100 mm Hg
    2. ECG changes (on ETT)
    3. Echo features of LV enlargement or reduced function

  Ideally replace the valve prior to significant left ventricular dilatation and dysfunction

PROGNOSIS
- Asymptomatic with EF >50% – 1% mortality at 5 years
- Symptomatic and all three criteria present – 65% mortality at 3 years

Mitral stenosis

This patient has been complaining of reduced exercise tolerance. Examine his heart and elucidate the cause of his symptoms.

Clinical signs

- Malar flush
- Irregular pulse if AF is present
- Tapping apex (palpable first heart sound)
- Left parasternal heave if pulmonary hypertension is present or enlarged left atrium
- Auscultation:

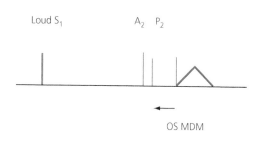

Loud first heart sound. Opening snap (OS) of mobile mitral leaflets opening followed by a mid-diastolic murmur (MDM), which is best heard at the apex, in the left lateral position in expiration with the bell. Presystolic accentuation of the MDM occurs if the patient is in sinus rhythm.

- **Severe if** OS occurs nearer A_2 (left atrial pressure higher, opens MV earlier) or is inaudible (fixed leaflets) and the MDM is longer
- **Complications:**
  - **Pulmonary hypertension and right heart failure:** tricuspid regurgitation, right ventricular heave, loud P_2, sacral and pedal oedema.
  - **Pulmonary oedema**
  - **Endocarditis**
  - **Embolic complications:** stroke risk is high if mitral stenosis + AF

Discussion

CAUSES

- Congenital
  - Rare
- **Acquired**
  - **Rheumatic** (commonest)
  - Senile degeneration
  - Large mitral leaflet vegetation from endocarditis (mitral 'plop' and late diastolic murmur)

DIFFERENTIAL DIAGNOSIS

- Left atrial myxoma
- Austin–Flint murmur

INVESTIGATION

- **ECG:** p-mitrale (broad, bifid) and atrial fibrillation
- **CXR:** enlarged left atrium (splayed of carina), calcified valve, pulmonary oedema
- **TTE/TOE:** valve area (<1.0 cm², gradient >10 mm Hg is severe), cusp mobility, calcification and left atrial thrombus, right ventricular failure and pulmonary hypertension (>50 mm Hg is severe)
- **Cardiac catheter:** coronary anatomy, right heart pressures

MANAGEMENT

- **Medical:** + AF: rate control and oral anticoagulants, diuretics
- **Mitral valvuloplasty:** if pliable, non-calcified with minimal regurgitation and no left atrial thrombus
- **Surgery:** closed mitral valvotomy (without opening the heart) or open valvotomy (requiring cardiopulmonary bypass) or valve replacement

PROGNOSIS

- Latent asymptomatic phase 15–20 years
- NYHA >II – 50% mortality at 5 years

RHEUMATIC FEVER

- Immunological cross-reactivity between Group A β-haemolytic streptococcal infection, e.g. *Streptococcus pyogenes* and valve tissue
- **Duckett–Jones diagnostic criteria:** proven β-haemolytic streptococcal infection diagnosed by throat swab, rapid antigen detection test (RADT), anti-streptolysin O titre (ASOT) or clinical scarlet fever **plus** 2 major or 1 major and 2 minor:

Major	Minor
Chorea	Raised ESR
Erythema marginatum	Raised WCC
Subcutaneous nodules	Arthralgia
Polyarthritis	Previous rheumatic fever
Carditis	Pyrexia
	Prolonged PR interval

- **Treatment:** Rest, high-dose aspirin and penicillin
- **Prophylaxis:**
  - Primary prevention: penicillin V (or clindamycin) for 10 days
  - Secondary prevention: penicillin V for about 5–10 years

Mitral incompetence

This patient has been short of breath and tired. Please examine his cardiovascular system.

Clinical signs
- Scars: lateral thoracotomy (valvotomy)
- Pulse: AF, small volume
- Apex: displaced and volume loaded
- Palpation: thrill at apex
- Auscultation:

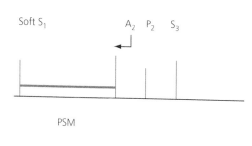

Soft S_1 A_2 P_2 S_3

PSM

High-pitched pan-systolic murmur (PSM) loudest at the apex radiating to the axilla. Loudest in expiration. Wide splitting of A_2P_2 due to the earlier closure of A_2 because the LV empties sooner. S_3 is low pitched and indicates rapid ventricular filling from LA and excludes significant mitral stenosis. Cadence: Slosh S_1, -ing S_2, -in S_3!

- **Severe if:** holosystolic (may be late systolic if mild), not murmur intensity
- **Complications:**
  - **Atrial fibrillation:** LA enlargement
  - **Pulmonary oedema:** increased LA pressure and LV failure
  - **Pulmonary hypertension**
  - **Endocarditis**
  - **Associated cardiac lesions**, e.g. ASD

Discussion

CAUSES
- Congenital (association between cleft mitral valve and primum ASD)
- Acquired:

	Acute	Chronic
Valve leaflets	Bacterial endocarditis	Myxomatous degeneration (prolapse)
		Rheumatic
		Connective tissue diseases
		Fibrosis (fenfluramine/pergolide)
Valve annulus		Dilated left ventricle (functional MR)
		Calcification
Chordae/papillae	Rupture	Infiltration, e.g. amyloid
		Fibrosis (post-MI/trauma)

INVESTIGATION
- **ECG:** p-mitrale, atrial fibrillation and previous infarction (Q waves)
- **CXR:** cardiomegaly, enlargement of the left atrium and pulmonary oedema
- **TTE/TOE:** size/density of MR jet, LV dilatation and reduced EF (severity) as well as cause: prolapse, vegetations, torn chordae or ruptured papillae (flail), fibrotic restriction and infarction, LV size; associated lesions: ASD, pulmonary pressure, RV size and function, TR
- **Cardiac MRI:** volume of MR (severity), LV dimensions and infarct (LGE)
- **Cardiac catheter:** right heart pressure

MANAGEMENT
- Medical
  - Anticoagulation for AF or embolic complications
  - Diuretic, β-blocker and ACE inhibitors
- **Percutaneous:**
  - Transcatheter edge-to-edge repair (TEER) – if high surgical risk and refractory heart failure symptoms despite optimal medical therapy
  - Lesion: degenerative MVP (primary or degenerative) and possibly also selected cases of functional MR
- **Surgical**
  - Valve repair (preferable) with annuloplasty ring or valve replacement
  - Aim to operate when symptomatic, prior to severe LV dilatation and dysfunction

PROGNOSIS
- Often asymptomatic for >10 years
- Symptomatic – 25% mortality at 5 years

Mitral valve prolapse
- Common (2–3%), especially young, lean, tall women
- Myxomatous degeneration – thick/long redundant mitral leaflets that fail to co-apt
- Associated with connective tissue disease, e.g. Marfan's (90%), SVT and HOCM
- Often asymptomatic and benign, but may present with chest pain, syncope and palpitations
- Rarely may present with severe MR, AF, SCD, emboli or endocarditis
- Auscultation:

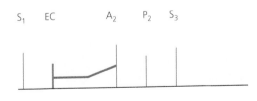

S_1 EC A_2 P_2 S_3

Mid-systolic ejection click (EC). Pan-systolic murmur that gets louder up to A_2. Murmur is accentuated (earlier EC and longer PSM) by standing from a squatting position or during the straining phase of the Valsalva manoeuvre, which reduces LV filling.

Tricuspid incompetence

Examine this patient's cardiovascular system. He has been complaining of abdominal discomfort.

Clinical signs

- Raised JVP with giant CV waves
- Thrill left sternal edge
- Auscultation:

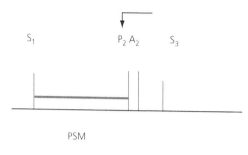

PSM

High-pitched pan-systolic murmur (PSM) loudest at the tricuspid area (lower left sternal edge) in inspiration, radiating to right sternal border. Reverse split second heart sound due to rapid RV emptying and early closure of P_2. Right ventricular rapid filling may give an S_3.

- RV failure: Pulsatile liver, ascites and peripheral oedema
- Pulmonary hypertension: RV heave and loud P_2

Discussion

CAUSES

- **Congenital: Ebstein's anomaly** (atrialization of the right ventricle and TR)
- **Acquired:**
  - ○ **Acute: Infective endocarditis** (IV drug user) – needle marks
  - ○ **Chronic:**
    - ○ **Functional** (commonest – dilated RV and annulus due to left heart disease)
    - ○ **Implantable device leads:** splinting tricuspid leaflet open – pacemaker scar
    - ○ **Carcinoid** – craggy liver
    - ○ **Rheumatic –** with other valve lesions, e.g. MS

INVESTIGATION

- **ECG:** p-pulmonale (large, peaked), AF and RV strain: large R-wave V1, TWI V1–3
- **CXR:** double right heart border (enlarged right atrium)
- **TTE:** TR jet, RV dilatation

MANAGEMENT

- **Medical:** diuretics, β-blockers, ACE inhibitors and support stockings for oedema
- **Percutaneous:** TEER, tricuspid annulus reduction (experimental)
- **Surgical:** valve repair/annuloplasty if medical treatment fails

Pulmonary stenosis
Examine this patient's cardiovascular system. He has had swollen ankles.

Clinical signs
- Raised JVP with giant A waves
- Left parasternal heave
- Thrill in the pulmonary area
- Auscultation:

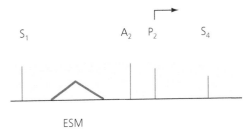

S_1 A_2 P_2 S_4

ESM

High-pitched ejection systolic murmur (ESM) heard loudest in the pulmonary area in inspiration. Widely split second heart sounds, due to a delay in RV emptying.

- Right ventricular failure: ascites and peripheral oedema
- **Severe if:** inaudible P_2, longer murmur duration obscuring A_2

ASSOCIATIONS
- **Tetralogy of Fallot:** PS, VSD, overriding aorta and RVH (sternotomy scar)
- **Noonan's syndrome:** phenotypically like Turner's syndrome but male sex
- Other murmurs: functional TR and VSD

Discussion
INVESTIGATION
- **ECG:** p-pulmonale, RVH and RBBB
- **CXR:** oligaemic lung fields and large right atrium
- **TTE:** severity (pressure gradient), RV function and associated cardiac lesions
- **Cardiac catheterization:** to guide intervention

MANAGEMENT
- Pulmonary valvotomy – if gradient >70 mm Hg or there is RV failure
- Percutaneous pulmonary valve implantation (PPVI)
- Surgical repair/replacement

Carcinoid syndrome
- Gut primary with liver metastasis secreting 5-HT into the bloodstream
- Toilet symptoms: diarrhoea, wheeze and flushing!
- Right heart valve fibrosis: "TIPS" - Tricuspid Insufficiency and Pulmonary Stenosis.
- Rarely a bronchogenic primary tumour or a right-to-left shunt can release 5-HT into the systemic circulation and cause left-sided valve fibrosis
- **Treatment:** long-acting somatostatin analogue and cytoreduction (ablation, embolization, surgical resection)

Prosthetic valves: aortic and mitral

This patient has recently been treated for dyspnoea/chest pain/syncope. Please examine his cardiovascular system.

Clinical signs

- Audible prosthetic clicks (metal) on approach and scars on inspection

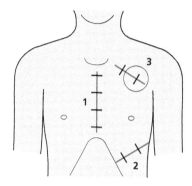

1 Midline sternotomy (CABG, AVR, MVR)
2 Lateral thoracotomy (MVR, mitral valvotomy, coarctation repair, BT shunt)
3 Subclavicular (pacemaker, ICD)

Also look in the wrist and groins for angiography scars/bruising and legs for saphenous vein harvest used in bypass grafts.

- Auscultation: don't panic!
  - **Aortic valve replacement:**

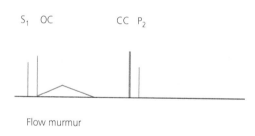

S_1 OC   CC P_2

Flow murmur

A metal prosthetic closing click (CC) is heard instead of A_2. There may be an opening click (OC) and high-pitched ejection systolic flow murmur. A bioprosthetic valve often has normal heart sounds. Abnormal findings: AR; decreased intensity of the closing click (clot or vegetation).

  - **Mitral valve replacement:**

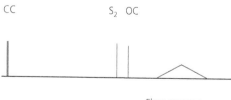

CC S_2 OC

Flow murmur

A metal prosthetic closing click is heard instead of S_1. An opening click may be heard in early diastole followed by a low-pitch diastolic rumble. Abnormal findings: MR; decreased intensity of the closing click.

- Anticoagulation: bruises (metal valve) and anaemia

Discussion

- Choice of surgical valve replacement

	For	Against	Indication
Metal	Durable	Warfarin	Young/on warfarin, e.g. for AF
Porcine	No warfarin	Less durable	Elderly/at risk of haemorrhage

- With the advent of percutaneous valve-in-valve TAVI for degenerative bioprosthetic valves in the mitral and aortic positions, fewer metallic surgical valves are being implanted
- Operative mortality: 1–5% depending on comorbidities and complexity of surgery

LATE COMPLICATIONS
- **Thromboembolus:** 1–2% per annum despite warfarin
- **Bleeding:** fatal 0.6%, major 3%, minor 7% per annum on warfarin
- **Bioprosthetic dysfunction and LVF:** usually within 10 years, can be treated percutaneously (valve-in-valve), paravalvular leak may be plugged percutaneously
- **Haemolysis:** mechanical red blood cell destruction against the metal valve or due to high-velocity paravalvular leak
- **Infective endocarditis:**
  - Early infective endocarditis (<2/12 post-op) can be due to *Staphylococcus epidermidis* from skin
  - Late infective endocarditis is often due to *Strep. viridans* by haematogenous spread
  - Prolonged high-dose IV antibiotics and a second valve replacement are usually required to treat this complication
  - Mortality of prosthetic valve endocarditis ranges from 20% to 80%
- **Atrial fibrillation:** particularly if MVR

Implantable devices

This patient has had syncope. Please examine his cardiovascular system.

Clinical signs
- Incisional scar in the infraclavicular position (may be abdominal)
- Palpation demonstrates a pacemaker
- Signs of heart failure: raised JVP, bibasal crackles and pedal oedema
- Medic alert bracelet
- **Complications:**
  - Acute/subacute:
    - Local infection: red/hot/tender/fluctuant/erosion
    - Pericardial effusion/tamponade
    - Pneumothorax
  - Chronic
    - Tricuspid regurgitation
    - Endocarditis

Discussion
NICE GUIDANCE
Implantable cardiac defibrillators (ICD):
- Subcutaneous (S-ICD) or transvenous (TV-ICD), the latter also delivers anti-tachycardia pacing (ATP) – improves mortality

PRIMARY PREVENTION
- MI > 4 weeks ago (NYHA no worse than class III):
  - LVEF <35% **and** non-sustained VT **and** positive EP study **or**
  - LVEF <30% **and** QRSd ≥120 ms
- Familial condition with high-risk SCD:
  - LQTS, ARVD, Brugada, HCM, complex congenital heart disease

SECONDARY PREVENTION (WITHOUT OTHER TREATABLE CAUSE)
- Cardiac arrest due to VT or VF **or**
- Haemodynamically compromising sustained VT **or**
- Sustained VT with LVEF <35% (not NYHA IV)

Cardiac resynchronization therapy (CRT) – biventricular pacemakers (BiV):
- Extra LV pacemaker lead via the coronary sinus – improves mortality/symptoms; may be considered if:
  - LVEF <35%
  - NYHA II–IV on optimal medical therapy
  - Sinus rhythm and QRSd ≥150 ms (if LBBB morphology may be >120 ms)

Constrictive pericarditis

This man has had previous mantle radiotherapy for lymphoma and has a chronic history of leg oedema, bloating and weight gain.

Clinical signs
- Predominantly right-sided heart failure:
  - o Raised JVP:
    - o Brief, dominant y-descent due to high RA pressures and an early rise in RV diastolic pressure due to poor pericardial compliance

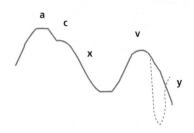

Jugular venous pressure waves. **a**, atrial systole; **c**, closure of tricuspid valve; **x**, movement of atrioventricular ring during ventricular systole; **v**, filling of the atrium; **y**, opening of the tricuspid valve.

  - o **Kussmaul's sign:** paradoxical increase in JVP on inspiration (may need to sit the patient at 90° rather than 45° to observe the JVP meniscus)
  - o **Pulsus paradoxus:**
    - o >10 mm Hg drop in systolic pressure in inspiration (not a true paradox as it normally decreases by 2–3 mm Hg!)
  - o Auscultation:
    - o Pericardial knock – it's not a knock but a high-pitched snap (audible, early S_3 due to rapid ventricular filling into a stiff pericardial sac)
  - o Ascites, hepatomegaly (congestion) and bilateral peripheral oedema
- Cause:
  - o **T**B: cervical lymphadenopathy
  - o **T**rauma (or surgery): sternotomy scar, post-MI
  - o **T**umour, **T**herapy (radio): radiotherapy tattoos, thoracotomy scar
  - o Connective **T**issue disease: rheumatoid hands, SLE signs

Discussion
INVESTIGATION
- **CXR:** pericardial calcification, old TB, sternotomy wires
- **Echo:** high acoustic signal from pericardium, septal bounce, reduced mitral flow velocity on Doppler during inspiration – ventricular interdependence
- **Cardiac catheter:**
  - o Dip and plateau of the diastolic wave form: square-root sign (due to high atrial pressures and poor ventricular compliance)
  - o Equalization of diastolic LV and RV, RA and LA pressures
  - o Ventricular interdependence: inspiration reduces LV filling/increases RV filling (and vice versa for expiration)
- **CT:** thickened pericardium ± calcification
- **Cardiac MRI:** thickened pericardium, fibrosis (LGE), early diastolic flattening of the septum, enlarged atria

PATHOPHYSIOLOGY
- Thickened, fibrous capsule reduces ventricular filling and 'insulates' the heart from intrathoracic pressure changes during respiration leading to **ventricular interdependence** – filling of one ventricle reduces the size and filling of the other

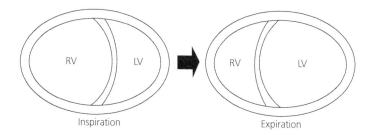

Inspiration   Expiration

Heart cavity in cross-section demonstrating septal motion during breathing indicating ventricular interdependence and constrictive physiology.

TREATMENT
- **Medical:** diuretics and fluid restriction
- **Surgical:** pericardiectomy
- Differentiating pericardial constriction from restrictive cardiomyopathy can be tricky, but observing ventricular interdependence (fluctuating LV/RV filling or MV/TV in-flow velocities during respiration) is highly diagnostic for constriction!

COMMON CONGENITAL DEFECTS

Atrial septal defect

This young woman complains of cough and occasional palpitations. Examine her cardiovascular system.

Clinical signs
- Raised JVP
- Pulmonary area thrill
- Auscultation:

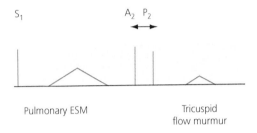

S_1 A_2 P_2

Pulmonary ESM   Tricuspid
                       flow murmur

Fixed split-second heart sounds that do not change with respiration. Pulmonary ejection systolic and mid-diastolic flow murmurs with large LTR shunts. There is no murmur from the ASD itself.

- **Signs of deterioration:**
  - Pulmonary hypertension: RV heave and loud P_2, + cyanosis and clubbing (Eisenmenger's: RTL shunt)
  - Congestive cardiac failure

Discussion

TYPES
- Primum associated with AVSD and cleft mitral valve) seen in Down's syndrome
- Secundum (commonest)

COMPLICATIONS
- Paradoxical embolus
- Atrial arrhythmias
- RV dilatation

INVESTIGATION
- **ECG:** RBBB + LAD (primum) or + RAD (secundum); atrial fibrillation
- **CXR:** small aortic knuckle, pulmonary plethora and double-heart border (enlarged RA)
- **TTE/TOE:** site, size and shunt calculation; amenability to closure – rims and partial anomalous pulmonary venous return (usually right upper pulmonary vein into RA)
- **Cardiac MRI:** shunt size and pulmonary venous anatomy, other defects
- **Right heart catheter:** shunt calculation (not always necessary)

MANAGEMENT
- Indications for closure:
  - Symptomatic: paradoxical systemic embolism, breathlessness
  - Significant shunt: Qp : Qs >1.5 : 1, RV dilatation
- Contraindication for closure:
  - Severe pulmonary hypertension and Eisenmenger's syndrome

CLOSURE
- Percutaneous closure device:
  - Secundum ASD only, no left atrial appendage thrombus or partial anomalous pulmonary venous drainage, adequate rim to anchor device
- Surgical patch repair

Ventricular septal defect
This patient has developed sudden shortness of breath. Examine his heart.

Clinical signs
- Thrill at the lower left sternal edge
- Auscultation:

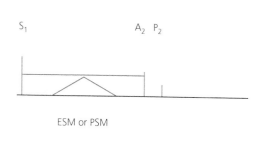

S_1 A_2 P_2

ESM or PSM

Usually, a high-pitched pansystolic murmur well localized at the left sternal edge with no radiation. No audible A_2. In large shunts an S_3 may be heard. Loudness does not correlate with size (maladie de Roger: loud murmur due to high-flow velocity through a small VSD). If Eisenmenger's develops the murmur often disappears as the gradient diminishes.

- **Also consider:**
  - Associated lesions: AR (subaortic VSD causes RCC prolapse), PDA (10%), Fallot's tetralogy and coarctation
  - Pulmonary hypertension: loud P_2 and RV heave + cyanosis and clubbing (Eisenmenger's)
  - Endocarditis

Discussion
CAUSES
- Congenital
- Acquired (traumatic, post-operative or post-MI)

INVESTIGATION
- **ECG:** conduction defect: BBB
- **CXR:** pulmonary plethora
- **TTE/TOE:** site, size, shunt calculation and associated lesions
- **Cardiac MRI:** site, size, shunt calculation and associated lesions
- **Cardiac catheter:** shunt size, pulmonary pressures, consideration of closure

MANAGEMENT
- **Conservative:** Small peri-membranous VSDs (commonest) often close spontaneously
- **Percutaneous:** Amplatzer® device
- **Surgical:** pericardial patch
- **Post-infarct VSD:**
  - 0.3% MI in PPCI era – bimodal: early (hours) subacute (3–5 days)
  - Decompensating LTR shunt: acute pulmonary oedema/cardiogenic shock
  - **Treatment:**
    - Mechanical circulatory support
    - Early closure with large patch to allow for further tissue loss and prevent dehiscence (late surgical closure after 7 days has better outcomes but is confounded by survivorship bias) or percutaneous closure device.
    - Heart transplant

ASSOCIATIONS WITH CONGENITAL VSD

1. Fallot's tetralogy

Clinical signs

- Right ventricular hypertrophy
- Overriding aorta
- VSD
- Pulmonary stenosis

- **Blalock-Taussig, Waterston and Potts shunts**
  - Partially corrects the Fallot's abnormality in infancy by anastomosing the subclavian artery (BT), ascending aorta (W) or descending aorta (P) to the pulmonary artery
  - Absent radial pulse (BT) and thoracic scars

- Other causes of an absent radial pulse:
  - **Acute:** embolism, aortic dissection, trauma, e.g. previous radial artery sheath
  - **Chronic:** atherosclerosis, coarctation, Takayasu's arteritis ('pulseless disease')

2. Coarctation

- A congenital narrowing of the aortic arch that is usually distal to the left subclavian artery and the ligamentum arteriosum (remnant of ductus) in adults

Clinical signs

- Hypertension in upper limbs
- Prominent upper body pulses, absent/weak femoral pulses, radio-femoral delay
- Heaving pressure-loaded apex
- Auscultation: usually systolic murmur from the coarctation (may be continuous murmur if well-developed collaterals) radiating through to the back. There is a loud A_2. There may be murmurs from associated lesions

Discussion

ASSOCIATIONS WITH COARCTATION
- **Cardiac:** VSD, bicuspid aortic valve and PDA
- **Non-cardiac:** Turner's syndrome and intracranial aneurysms

INVESTIGATION
- **ECG:** LVH (hypertension) and RBBB (associated VSD)
- **CXR:** rib notching, double aortic knuckle (pre- and post-stenotic dilatation – 'Figure 3 sign')
- **TTE:** increased aortic flow velocity on Doppler, associated lesions
- **CT/cardiac MRI:** defines anatomy for repair and associated lesions

MANAGEMENT
- Percutaneous: endovascular aortic repair (EVAR)
- Surgical: Dacron patch aortoplasty
- Long-term anti-hypertensive therapy (aortopathy and hypertension often persist)
- Long-term follow-up/surveillance with MRA: late aneurysms and recoarctation

3. Patent ductus arteriosus (PDA)

- Continuity between the aorta and pulmonary trunk with LTR shunt (very rare in adults)
- Risk factor: rubella

Clinical signs
- Collapsing pulse
- Thrill left second intercostal space
- Thrusting apex beat
- Auscultation: loud continuous 'machinery murmur' loudest below the left clavicle in systole

Discussion
COMPLICATIONS
- Eisenmenger's syndrome (5%)
- Endocarditis

MANAGEMENT
- Close surgically or plug percutaneously

Hypertrophic (obstructive) cardiomyopathy

This young man has complained of palpitations while playing football. Examine his cardiovascular system.

Clinical signs

- Jerky pulse character
- Double apical impulse (palpable atrial and ventricular contraction)
- Thrill at the lower left sternal edge
- Auscultation:

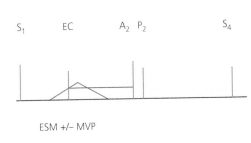

S_1 EC A_2 P_2 S_4

ESM +/– MVP

Ejection systolic murmur (ESM) at the lower left sternal edge that radiates throughout the precordium. A fourth heart sound (S_4) is present due to blood hitting a hypertrophied stiff LV during atrial systole. Dynamic ESM accentuated by reducing LV volume (LVOT becomes narrower), e.g. standing from squatting or during a strain phase of Valsalva (opposite to aortic valve stenosis).

- There may be associated mitral valve prolapse (MVP) (see Mitral Incompetence)
- There may be features of Friedreich's ataxia or myotonic dystrophy (see Neurology section)

Discussion

INVESTIGATION

- **ECG:** LVH with strain (deep T-wave inversion across precordial leads)
- **CXR:** often normal
- **TTE:** asymmetrical septal hypertrophy and systolic anterior motion of the anterior mitral leaflet across the LVOT due to misalignment of septal papillary muscle, LVOT gradient (rest/exercise or dobutamine stress)
- **Cardiac MRI:** identifies apical HCM more reliably than TTE, detects fibrosis (LGE)
- **Cardiac catheterization:** LVOT gradient accentuated by a ventricular ectopic or pharmacological stress, identification of septals
- **Genetic tests:** sarcomeric proteins mutation

DIFFERENTIAL DIAGNOSIS OF LVH

- Athletic heart
- Hypertensive heart disease
- HOCM
- Anderson–Fabry disease
- Cardiac amyloidosis

MANAGEMENT

- **Asymptomatic:**
  - Avoidance of strenuous exercise, dehydration and vasodilators
- Symptomatic and LVOT gradient >30 mm Hg:
  - β-Blockers and verapamil: lower heart rate – increasing diastolic time to fill stiff LV and negative inotropic agents reducing the force of LVOT compression
  - Cardiac myosin-inhibitors: mavacamten – negative inotrope (monitor LVEF with echo)
  - Pacemaker – altered ventricular electrical activation can relieve LVOT obstruction
  - Alcohol septal ablation or surgical myomectomy for persistent symptoms despite medical therapy (risk of pacemaker)

- Rhythm disturbance/high-risk SCD
  - ICD

- Refractory:
  - Heart transplantation

- Genetic counselling of first-degree relatives (autosomal dominant inheritance)

PROGNOSIS

- Annual mortality rate in adults is 2.5%
- Poor prognosis factors (indications for ICD):
  - Young age at diagnosis
  - Syncope
  - Documented VT or cardiac arrest
  - Family history of sudden cardiac death
  - Septal thickness ≥30 mm
  - 'Burnt-out' LV (reduced LVEF and fibrosis)

Heart failure

This middle-aged man has complained of fatigue, breathlessness and ankle swelling. Examine his cardiovascular system.

Clinical signs

- Raised JVP
- Displaced and hyperkinetic apex
- Auscultation: murmurs (e.g. functional MR and TR) and an S_3 gallop (if decompensated), loud P_2 if associated pulmonary hypertension
- Bibasal crackles and peripheral oedema

Discussion

CAUSES

- Inherited
- Acquired: **'SO DILATED'**
  - **S**tructural heart disease (valvular, congenital)
  - **O**besity
  - **D**rugs, e.g. anti-cancer therapy especially anthracyclines, **D**ystrophy
  - **Ischaemia (commonest), I**nfection, e.g. viral, **I**nfiltration, **I**nflammation
  - **L**iver and kidney disease
  - **A** baby (post-partum cardiomyopathy), **A**rrhythmias
  - **T**oxins (mercury and cobalt), **T**hyroid disease
  - **E**tOH, **E**levated BP
  - **D**iabetes

INVESTIGATION

- **ECG:** ischaemic changes, LBBB, AF
- **CXR:** increased CTR, interstitial (Kerley B/septal lines) and pulmonary 'bat-wing pattern' oedema
- **TTE:** LV size and function, associated lesions
- **Cardiac catheter:** LVEDP and coronary patency
- **Cardiac MRI:** LV size and function; aetiology, e.g. myocarditis – mid-wall LGE; infarction – subendocardial/full-wall thickness LGE

TREATMENT

- Treat cause (if known)
- Medical:
  - Fluid and salt restriction and diuretics
  - Four pillars: β-blocker, ACE inhibitor (ARB/ARNI), MRA, SGLT2 inhibitor
  - Thromboprophylaxis when hospitalized (no evidence supports routine use)
- Device:
  - ICD/CRT
- Surgery:
  - Volume reduction surgery – improving LVEDP–stroke volume relationship (Frank–Starling curves) and reducing LV wall stress
  - LVAD
  - Heart transplantation – donation after brain death (DBD) or donation after cardiac death/irreversible cessation of circulation (DCD) aided by ex vivo cardiac reanimation 'heart in a box' to expand the donor pool
- **Indications for heart transplantation:**
  - Severely impaired LV systolic function, HCM, intractable VT or angina
  - NYHA III or IV despite optimal medical therapy
  - CRT/ICD or CRT-D implanted
  - Poor prognosis:

- CPET: VO$_2$ max <14 ml/kg/min
- Markedly elevated BNP or NT-proBNP
- Seattle Heart Failure Model: 1 yr mortality >20%
- Cardiac cachexia
- Refractory cardiogenic shock despite mechanical support and inotropes (urgent)
- **Reasons to be turned down for cardiac transplantation in the UK:**
  - **Absolute contraindication:**
    - Age >65 and with another serious health condition
    - Sepsis and active infections
    - Active incurable malignancy (except local, non-melanoma skin cancer)
    - Psychosocial factors: continued smoking, EtOH and drug abuse; mental health problems; **poor compliance with immunosuppression**
    - Irreversible pulmonary hypertension/high PVR: **RVF of a transplanted heart**
  - **Relative contraindication:**
    - High BMI >32 kg/m^2
    - Diabetes with end organ damage
    - Severe peripheral or cerebrovascular disease
    - Severe lung or kidney disease
    - Severe osteoporosis
    - HIV/Hep B and C
- **Change in UK law – presumed consent for donor organs:**
  - Also known as 'opt-out' system; unless the deceased has expressed a wish in life not to be an organ donor then consent will be assumed

Neurology

Clinical mark sheet

Clinical skill	Satisfactory	Unsatisfactory
Physical examination	Correct, thorough, fluent, systematic, professional	Incorrect technique, omits, unsystematic, hesitant
Identifying physical signs	Identifies correct signs Does not find signs that are not present	Misses important signs Finds signs that are not present
Differential diagnosis	Constructs sensible differential diagnosis	Poor differential, fails to consider the correct diagnosis
Clinical judgement	Sensible and appropriate management plan	Inappropriate management Unfamiliar with management
Maintaining patient welfare	Respectful, sensitive Ensures comfort, safety and dignity	Causes physical or emotional discomfort Jeopardizes patient safety

Cases for PACES, Fourth Edition. Stephen Hoole, Andrew Fry and Rachel Davies.
© 2025 John Wiley & Sons Ltd. Published 2025 by John Wiley & Sons Ltd.

Neurology exam – general advice

Neurological examination requires two steps: (a) lesion localisation, *then* (b) knowing the differential diagnosis at each location. Some signs (e.g. pronator drift, extensor plantars) are far more robust than others (e.g. reduced sensation or reduced tone) – weight your examination findings accordingly.

Pertinent parts of the examination to localize the lesion

Learn a thorough routine, but cover the signs localizing the most frequent scenarios early.

CRANIAL NERVES

Start by systematically inspecting:

- **Face** – look for flattened nasolabial fold (most subtle sign of upper motor neurone (UMN) or lower motor neurone (LMN) facial weakness), while additional weakness of eye closure (orbicularis oculi) or eyebrow elevation (frontalis) indicates LMN
- **Eyes** – seek strabismus, anisocoria and ptosis (bilateral ptosis is missed unless explicitly sought)

If nothing found on inspection, then the most likely scenarios are visual field defects or abnormal eye movements (ophthalmoplegia or nystagmus).

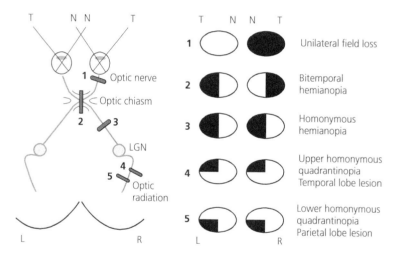

Visual field defects. N, nasal; T, temporal (field).

LIMB EXAMINATION

- First inspect; then examine pronator drift and finger–nose testing (arm exam) or gait ± Romberg's test – ability to maintain erect posture for 60 seconds with eyes closed (leg exam).
- **Systematically inspect:** wasting (usually LMN; rarely disuse from UMN), fasciculations (LMN) or rest tremor (Parkinsonism)
  - ○ Proximal wasting (uncommon):
    - ○ Arms: deltoid
    - ○ Legs: quadriceps
  - ○ **Distal wasting** (common)
    - ○ Arms: thenar eminence (median nerve lesions), hypothenar eminence and dorsal guttering (ulnar nerve lesions)

- o Legs: pes cavus (indicates motor polyneuropathy during development, especially HMSN or Friedreich's ataxia), tibialis anterior
- o Interpretation:
  - o Bilateral wasting indicates (motor) polyneuropathy (usually symmetrical) or anterior horn cell disease or mononeuritis multiplex (both usually asymmetrical)
  - o Unilateral wasting indicates mononeuropathy or radiculopathy
- o **Fasciculations:**
  - o Without weakness = benign
  - o If weak too, then caused by any LMN lesion, though in general if widespread = MND (or rarely syringomyelia) while focal fasciculations = radiculopathy
- • **Pronator drift:**
  - o Unilateral indicates contralateral brain hemisphere lesion
  - o Bilateral usually indicates cervical cord or brainstem; less commonly bilateral hemisphere
  - o Also seek postural tremor while hands outstretched
- • **Intention tremor** (during finger-nose testing): indicates ipsilateral cerebellar lesion
- • **Gait:** instruct to walk normally away (if safe to do so); then heel-to-toe coming back (to uncover subtle ataxia)
  - o **Circumduction/ hemiplegic/spastic** (as increased tone forces plantar flexion):
    - o Unilateral = contralateral brain lesion
    - o Bilateral = spinal cord (rarely = brainstem or bilateral hemisphere)
  - o **High stepping/neuropathic** (to overcome distal weakness with low tone)
    - o Unilateral = mononeuropathy (common peroneal) or radiculopathy (L5)
    - o Bilateral = (motor) polyneuropathy
  - o **Waddling/myopathic = myopathy**
  - o **Ataxic/staggering**
    - o Cerebellar (Romberg's negative)
    - o Sensory ataxia (i.e. reduced joint position sense from cord lesion or polyneuropathy – Romberg's positive)
- • **Power:** use gravity, e.g. raise leg off bed or raise arms, getting out of chair
  - o Weakness from UMN lesions has a **characteristic 'pyramidal' distribution:** extensors are usually weaker than flexors in the upper limbs and vice versa in the lower limbs
- • **Tone and reflexes:** assess tone by rotating wrist (for rigidity) and supinating/pronating elbow (for spasticity); clonus indicates severe spasticity
  - o **Spasticity:** velocity dependent (subtle spasticity only felt with fast movements); this is a UMN sign
  - o **Rigidity:** not velocity dependent, usually has tremor superimposed causing cogwheel rigidity; indicates Parkinsonism

		Tone	Reflexes	Plantars
UMN: Brain, spinal cord	Everything up	⇑	⇑	⇑
LMN: Cauda equina, nerve root, nerve	Everything down	⇓	⇓	⇓
Muscle/ neuromuscular	Normal	N	N	N

LOCALISE THE LESION

Location	Signs	Distribution	Other pointers	Common causes
Brain	UMN	Unilateral		Stroke, tumour, MS (abscess, subdural)
Spinal cord	UMN	Bilateral	Sensory level Bladder/bowel	Stroke, tumour, MS, disc/spondylosis (abscess)
Cauda equina	LMN	Bilateral	Sensory level Bladder/bowel Back pain ++	Disc/spondylosis, tumour
Nerve root (radiculopathy)	LMN	Unilateral	Dermatomal and myotomal	Disc/spondylosis, tumour
Peripheral nerve (polyneuropathy)	LMN	Bilateral	Distal (glove and stocking) though GBS/ CIDP also proximal	**Hours to days of progression** GBS, porphyria, diabetic amyotrophy, lead poisoning (all predominantly motor) **Months to years of progression** Paraprotein (60% IgM) Paraneoplastic (anti-hu or anti-CV2) Infection (HIV, Lyme, leprosy) Immune (CIDP) Metabolic (DM, renal failure, deficiencies – B_1, B_{12}, pyridoxine) **Years to decades of progression** **HMSN (aka CMT)**[m]
Peripheral nerve (mononeuropathy)	LMN	Unilateral	Specific nerve distribution	Entrapment at vulnerable sites; may be exacerbated in systemic conditions, e.g. pregnancy, DM, RA
Neuromuscular junction	Normal	Bilateral	Proximal Motor only Fatigable (MG) Ptosis (MG)	**Myasthenia gravis** (reduced power with use) Rarer: Lambert–Eaton myasthenic syndrome (increased power with use) – dry mouth Botulism (canned food, soil, IV drug use) – sialorrhoea and mydriasis
Myopathy	Normal	Bilateral	Proximal Motor only Not fatigable	Toxic: drugs (statins, steroids), EtOH Metabolic: osteomalacia, hypo/ hyperthyroid Infections: HIV, hepatitis B and C, influenza, enterovirus Inflammatory: polymyositis, dermatomyositis, inclusion body myositis Inherited: Duchenne/Becker, myotonic, FSHD, limb-girdle Rare: congenital, metabolic, channelopathy

EXCEPTIONS TO THE RULE

- Occasionally bilateral UMN signs occur from bilateral brain lesions
- Unilateral UMN signs can occur from a hemicord syndrome, e.g. characteristically **Brown-Séquard:** ipsilateral loss of power and joint position sense/vibration (from corticospinal tract and dorsal column damage, respectively, both of which decussate in the medulla) and contralateral pinprick loss (from spinothalamic tract damage, which decussates at or near the nerve root entry level)
- Rarely, systemic conditions can pick off random nerves, giving an asymmetrical pattern of LMN features (sensory and motor), e.g. a left radial neuropathy and a right ulnar. This is called **mononeuritis multiplex**. The causes include diabetes mellitus, SLE, RA, vasculitis (e.g. polyarteritis nodosum and Churg–Strauss) and infection (e.g. HIV)
- **Combined UMN and LMN features** indicate:
  - motor neurone disease (motor only)
  - cervical myeloradiculopathy (motor, often sensory or sphincter involvement too)
  - diseases affecting the central and peripheral nervous system (Friedreich's ataxia, vitamin B_{12} deficiency (subacute combined degeneration of the cord plus peripheral neuropathy)

Dystrophia myotonica

This man complains of worsening weakness in his hands. Please examine him.

Clinical signs

FACE
- Myopathic facies: long, thin and expressionless
- Wasting of facial muscles and sternocleidomastoid
- Bilateral ptosis
- Frontal balding
- Dysarthria: due to myotonia of tongue and pharynx

HANDS
- **Myotonia:** 'Grip my hand, now let go' (may be obscured by profound weakness); 'Screw up your eyes tightly shut, now open them'
- **Wasting** and **weakness** of distal muscles (especially finger flexors) with areflexia
- **Percussion myotonia:** percuss thenar eminence and watch for involuntary thumb flexion

ADDITIONAL SIGNS
- Cataracts
- Cardiomyopathy, brady- and tachyarrhythmias (look for pacemaker scar)
- Diabetes
- Testicular atrophy
- Dysphagia (ask about swallowing)

Discussion

GENETICS
- Dystrophia myotonica can be categorised as type 1 (common) or 2 (rare) depending on the underling genetic defect:
  - DM1: expansion of CTG trinucleotide repeat sequence within *DMPK* gene on chromosome 19
  - DM2: expansion of CCTG tetranucleotide repeat sequence within *ZNF9* gene on chromosome 3
- **Genetic anticipation:** worsening severity of the condition and earlier age of presentation within successive generations. Seen in DM1; also occurs in Huntington's disease (autosomal dominant) and Friedreich's ataxia (autosomal recessive)
- Both DM1 and DM2 are autosomal dominant
- DM1 usually presents in 20s–40s (DM2 later), but can be very variable depending on number of triplet repeats

DIAGNOSIS
- Clinical features
- EMG: 'dive-bomber' potentials
- Genetic testing

MANAGEMENT
- Affected individuals die prematurely of respiratory and cardiac complications
- Weakness is major problem – no treatment
- Mexiletine (or phenytoin) may help myotonia
- Advise against general anaesthetic (high risk of respiratory/cardiac complications)

Common causes of ptosis

Bilateral	Unilateral
Myotonic dystrophy (not fatigable)	IIIrd nerve palsy – pupil enlarged (surgical) or normal (medical)
Myasthenia gravis (fatigable)	Horner's syndrome – pupil small
Congenital	

Cerebellar syndrome

This 37-year-old woman has noticed increasing problems with her coordination. Please examine her and suggest a diagnosis.

Clinical signs ('DANISH')

- **D**ysdiadochokinesis
- **A**taxia
- **N**ystagmus
- **I**ntention tremor
- **S**canning dysarthria
- **H**ypotonia/hyporeflexia

- Cerebellar hemisphere lesions produce ipsilateral *limb* signs
- Cerebellar vermis (midline) lesions cause *truncal* ataxia (impairing sitting and walking) balance but no limb ataxia
- Nystagmus reflects cerebellar or peripheral (vestibular) lesions. By convention, the direction of the fast phase determines the direction of nystagmus:
  - Cerebellar lesion: fast-phase direction *changes* with changing direction of gaze
  - Vestibular nucleus/VIII nerve lesions (usually BPPV or vestibular neuritis): fast-phase direction *does not change* with changing direction of gaze, and fast phase is **away from** the side of the lesion and maximal on looking **away from** the lesion

Discussion

CAUSES ('PASTRIES')

- **P**araneoplastic cerebellar syndrome
- **A**lcohol – Wernicke's encephalopathy (subacute) or cerebellar degeneration (chronic)
- **S**clerosis – MS
- **T**umour – posterior fossa SOL
- **R**ecessive (e.g. Friedreich's, ataxia telangiectasia) or dominant (spinocerebellar ataxias)
- **I**atrogenic – phenytoin toxicity
- **E**ndocrine – hypothyroidism
- **S**troke – cerebellar (or brainstem) vascular event

Aetiological clues

Clue	Cause
Internuclear ophthalmoplegia, spasticity, female, younger age	MS
Optic atrophy	MS and Friedrich's ataxia
Clubbing, tar-stained fingers, radiotherapy burn	Bronchial carcinoma
Stigmata of liver disease, unkempt appearance	EtOH
Neuropathy	EtOH and Friedreich's ataxia
Gingival hypertrophy	Phenytoin

Multiple sclerosis

This 30-year-old woman complains of double vision and incoordination with previous episodes of weakness. Please perform a neurological examination.

Clinical signs (depend on site of plaques)

- **Inspection:** wheelchair; catheter (if spinal plaque)
- **Cranial nerves:** any UMN signs. Characteristically internuclear ophthalmoplegia (often bilateral), RAPD/optic disc atrophy/reduced visual acuity (if optic neuritis)
- **Limbs:** Sensory and UMN signs from brain or spinal cord plaques
- **Cerebellar:** 'DANISH' (see Cerebellar Syndrome)
- **Internuclear ophthalmoplegia:** Indicates a lesion in the (heavily myelinated) medial longitudinal fasciculus (MLF), which connects the paramedian pontine reticular formation (PPRF) and VIth nerve nucleus on one side to the IIIrd nerve nucleus on the other, enabling conjugate eye movements. MS is the most common cause. Lesions are often bilateral in MS and unilateral in stroke.

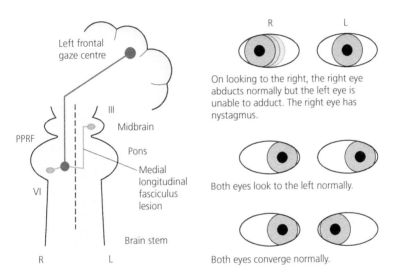

On looking to the right, the right eye abducts normally but the left eye is unable to adduct. The right eye has nystagmus.

Both eyes look to the left normally.

Both eyes converge normally.

Left internuclear ophthalmoplegia

Discussion

DIAGNOSTIC CRITERIA

- Requires dissemination in **time** and **space** (conventionally two distinct relapses in different CNS locations)
- McDonald criteria allow MS to be diagnosed after a single attack using paraclinical tests
- Dissemination in space is fulfilled if there are lesions in at least two predefined locations, and dissemination in time may be fulfilled with either (a) MRI (enhancing (i.e. <3 months old) and non-enhancing (>3 months old) lesions; or new lesions on a second MRI; *or* (b) oligoclonal bands in the CSF

SUBTYPES

- Relapse-onset in 85% – relapsing-remitting (RRMS), though convert to secondary progressive (SPMS) after median 15 years
- 15% are progressive from onset – primary progressive (PPMS)

CAUSE
- Incompletely understood
- A third of disease risk is genetic (>200 alleles, especially HLA-DRB1*15:01, but <1% carriers develop MS)
- Another third reflects environmental risks (increasing latitude, vitamin D deficiency, Epstein–Barr virus, smoking)
- The remaining third reflects interactions between genes and environment

INVESTIGATION
- **Clinical diagnosis plus:**
  - CSF: oligoclonal IgG bands
  - MRI: periventricular, juxtacortical, infratentorial, cortical or spinal cord lesions
  - Visual evoked potentials (VEPs): delayed velocity but normal amplitude (indicates optic neuritis)
- **Other clinical features:**
  - Higher mental function: fatigue, depression, cognitive
  - Autonomic: urinary retention/incontinence, impotence and bowel problems

  - **Uthoff's phenomenon:** worsening of symptoms with heat (e.g. bath) or exercise
  - **Lhermitte's sign:** shock-like pain down spine/limbs on neck flexion (due to cervical cord plaques)

TREATMENT
- **Multidisciplinary approach:** MS-specialist nurse, physiotherapist, occupational therapist, social worker and physician
- **Disease-modifying treatments:**
  - For RRMS, over a dozen drugs reduce relapses by a third (e.g. interferon-β), by half (e.g. fingolimod) or by 80–90% (monoclonal antibodies, e.g. natalizumab). Also graded effects on disability and on delaying conversion to SPMS. But with growing efficacy comes greater toxicity
  - For early PPMS ocrelizumab (anti-CD20) modestly effective if active MRI scan
- **Symptomatic treatments:**
  - Methylprednisolone (oral/IV) shortens relapses but does not alter prognosis
  - Anti-spasmodics, e.g. baclofen
  - Gabapentin, pregabalin or amitriptyline (for neuropathic pain)
  - Laxatives and intermittent catheterization/oxybutynin for bowel/bladder disturbance

MS AND PREGNANCY
- Reduced relapse rate during pregnancy (but increased in postpartum period)
- Safe for foetus
- ~2% risk of MS in children of parent with MS

IMPAIRMENT, DISABILITY AND HANDICAP
- Arm paralysis is the **impairment**
- Inability to write is the **disability**
- Subsequent inability to work as an accountant is the **handicap**
- Occupational therapy aims to help minimize the disability and abolish the handicap of arm paresis

Stroke
Examine this patient's limbs neurologically and then proceed to examine anything else that you feel is important.

Clinical signs (depend on site of stroke)
- **Inspection:** walking aids, nasogastric tube or PEG tube, fixed deformities (flexed upper limbs and extended lower limbs)
- **Cranial nerves:** any UMN sign – often facial weakness, homonymous hemianopia
- **Speech:** dysarthria (spastic) or dysphasia – expressive dysphasia – Broca's area (frontal lobe); and/or receptive dysphasia – Wernicke's area (temporal lobe)
- **Limbs:** unilateral UMN signs (though first ~2 days may appear LMN) and reduced sensation
- **Cerebellar:** 'DANISH' (see Cerebellar Syndrome)
- **MRC grading of muscle power:**
  - 0, none
  - 1, flicker
  - 2, moves with gravity neutralized
  - 3, moves against gravity
  - 4, reduced power against resistance
  - 5, normal
- **Other signs:**
  - Offer to perform bedside swallow assessment
  - Higher cortical functions, e.g. sensory or visual inattention
  - **Cause:** irregular pulse (AF), BP, cardiac murmurs or carotid bruits (anterior circulation stroke). If headache at onset seek temporal tenderness (for giant cell arteritis) and Horner's syndrome (for carotid/vertebral dissection)
  - Neck scars from carotid endarterectomy

Discussion
DEFINITIONS
- **Stroke:** rapid-onset focal neurological deficit due to vascular lesion lasting >24 h
- **Transient ischaemic attack (TIA):** same but lasts <24 h (typically <30 min)

INVESTIGATION
- **Bloods:** FBC, CRP/ESR, glucose/HbA1c, lipids and renal function
- **ECG:** AF or previous infarction
- **CXR:** cardiomegaly or aspiration
- **CT head:** infarct or bleed, territory
- **MRI brain perfusion:** salvageable vs irreversibly infarcted brain tissue
- **24-hour ECG** (or inpatient telemetry during admission): paroxysmal arrhythmia (AF)
- **Echocardiogram**
- **Carotid Dopplers**
- Consider CT angiogram, MRI/A/V (dissection or venous sinus thrombosis in young patient), clotting screen (thrombophilia), vasculitis screen in young stroke

MANAGEMENT
- **Acute**
  - Thrombolysis with tPA (within 4.5 hours of acute ischaemic stroke)
  - Thrombectomy (interventional radiology) up to 24 h of acute ischaemic stroke (preferably within 6 h) if CTA shows proximal occlusion (internal carotid, MCA M1, basilar or vertebral)
  - Aspirin (300 mg od for first two weeks – clopidogrel if intolerant)
  - Referral to a specialist multidisciplinary stroke unit: physiotherapy, occupational therapy, speech and language therapy and specialist stroke rehabilitation nurses
  - DVT prophylaxis

- **Chronic**
  - Refer for carotid endarterectomy if anterior circulation stroke and >70% stenosis of ipsilateral internal carotid artery (consider if >50% stenosis)
  - Anticoagulation for cardiac thromboembolism if AF detected (not in acute phase)
  - Address cardiovascular risk factors
  - Nursing ± social care.
  - Driving restrictions: 1 month off if satisfactory recovery (1 month off post TIA too)

BAMFORD CLASSIFICATION OF STROKE (LANCET 1991)
- **Total anterior circulation stroke (TACS)**
  - **H**emiplegia (contralateral to the lesion)
  - **H**omonymous hemianopia (contralateral to the lesion)
  - **H**igher cortical dysfunction, e.g. dysphasia, dyspraxia and neglect
- **Partial anterior circulation stroke (PACS)**
  - 2/3 of the above
- **Lacunar stroke (LACS)**
  - Pure hemi-motor or sensory loss

Prognosis at 1 year (%)

	TACS	PACS	LACS
Dead	60	15	10
Dependent	35	30	30
Independent	5	55	60

LATERAL MEDULLARY (WALLENBERG) SYNDROME
- Most common brainstem stroke
- Due to occlusion of posterior inferior cerebellar artery (PICA)
- Variable presentation but frequently acute vertigo/vomiting plus Horner's syndrome
- Treated in the same way as other strokes

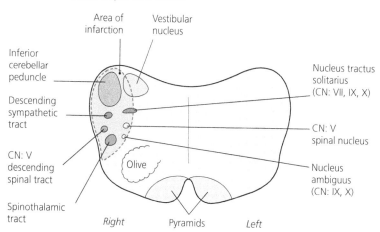

Brainstem structures affected by right-sided lesion

Clinical consequences of this lesion

Localization	Clinical sign(s)	Brainstem structure affected
Ipsilateral to lesion (e.g. on right with right-sided infarction)	Cerebellar signs	Inferior cerebellar peduncle
	Nystagmus	Vestibular nucleus
	Horner's syndrome	Descending sympathetic tract
	Palatal sensory loss and weakness	Nucleus ambiguus (CN IX and X)
	Loss of facial pain and temperature sensation	Trigeminal nerve (CN V) spinal nucleus and tract
Contralateral to lesion (e.g. on left with right-sided lesion)	Loss of limb pain and temperature sensation	Spinothalamic tract

Spastic legs (i.e. spinal cord lesion)

Examine this man's lower limbs neurologically. He has had difficulty in walking.

Clinical signs

- Wheelchair or walking sticks, catheter
- Bilateral UMN signs, sensory level (see neurological general exam advice)

ADDITIONAL SIGNS

- Search for features of common causes, e.g.:
  - ○ Multiple sclerosis, e.g. RAPD, internuclear ophthalmoplegia, cerebellar
  - ○ Scars or spinal deformity to suggest orthopaedic cause

Discussion

COMMON CAUSES

- Multiple sclerosis
- Spinal cord compression/myelopathy/trauma
- MND (no sensory signs)

RARE CAUSES

- Anterior spinal artery stroke: spinothalamic (pain/temperature) and corticospinal (weakness) tract loss with preservation of dorsal columns
- Inflammatory: neuromyelitis optica (seek evidence of optic neuritis), SLE, Sjögren's
- Syringomyelia
- Hereditary spastic paraplegia: spasticity exceeds weakness, positive family history
- B_{12} deficiency: subacute combined degeneration of the cord; also has neuropathy
- Friedreich's ataxia: also cerebellar signs, peripheral neuropathy (causing pes cavus)
- Parasagittal falx meningioma: compresses the (midline) leg motor cortex areas

CORD COMPRESSION

- **Emergency**
- **Causes:** disc, bone, tumour, abscess
- **Investigation of choice:** spinal MRI
- **Treatment:**
  - ○ Urgent surgical decompression
  - ○ Consider steroids and radiotherapy (for a malignant cause)

Lumbosacral root levels

L 1/2	Hip flexion	
L 2/3	Hip adduction	
L 3/4	Knee extension	**Knee jerk L 3/4**
L 4/5	Ankle dorsiflexion/inversion/eversion	
L 5/ S 1	Knee flexion	
	Hip extension	
S 1/2	Foot plantarflexion	**Ankle jerk S 1/2**

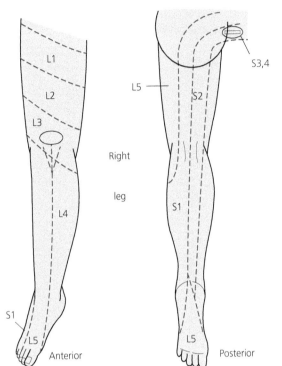

Right

leg

Anterior

Posterior

Lower limb dermatomes. Hints: L3 (knee); L4 (to the floor medially); S2, 3, 4 (keeps the faeces off the floor!).

Syringomyelia

Examine this patient's upper limbs neurologically. He has been complaining of numb hands.

Clinical signs

- Weakness and wasting of small muscles of the hand
- Loss of reflexes in the upper limbs
- Dissociated sensory loss in upper limbs and chest: loss of pain and temperature sensation (spinothalamic) with preservation of joint position and vibration sense (dorsal columns)
- Scars from painless burns
- Charcot joints: elbow and shoulder

Additional signs

- Pyramidal weakness in lower limbs with upgoing (extensor) plantars
- Kyphoscoliosis is common
- Horner's syndrome
- If syrinx extends into brain stem (syringobulbia) there may be cerebellar and lower cranial nerve signs

Discussion

- Syringomyelia is caused by a progressively expanding fluid-filled cavity (syrinx) within the cervical cord, typically spanning several levels

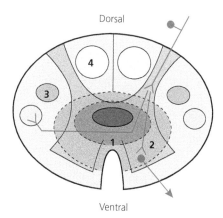

Syrinx expands ventrally affecting:

1. Decussating spinothalamic neurones producing segmental pain and temperature loss at the level of the syrinx.
2. Anterior horn cells producing segmental lower motor neurone weakness at the level of the syrinx.
3. Corticospinal tract producing upper motor neurone weakness below the level of the syrinx.

It usually spares the dorsal columns (4 – proprioception and vibration).

- The signs may be asymmetrical
- Frequently associated with an Arnold–Chiari malformation and spina bifida
- Investigation = spinal MRI

CHARCOT JOINT (NEUROPATHIC ARTHROPATHY)

- Painless deformity and destruction of a joint with new bone formation following repeated minor trauma secondary to loss of pain sensation
- The most important causes are:
  - Tabes dorsalis: hip and knee
  - Diabetes: foot and ankle
  - Syringomyelia: elbow and shoulder
- Treatment: bisphosphonates can help

Cervical roots

C 5	Shoulder abduction	
C 5/6	Elbow flexion and supination	**Biceps and supinator jerks C 5/6**
C 6/7	Elbow and wrist extension	**Triceps jerk C 7/8**
C 7	Finger extension	
C 8	Finger flexion	
T 1	Finger abduction	

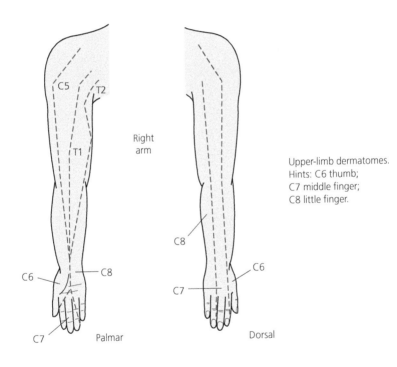

Right arm

Palmar

Dorsal

Upper-limb dermatomes.
Hints: C6 thumb;
C7 middle finger;
C8 little finger.

Motor neurone disease

This man complains of gradually increasing weakness. Please examine him neurologically.

Clinical signs (combination of UMN and LMN signs with preserved sensation)

- **Inspection:** wasting and fasciculation
- **Tone:** usually spastic but can be flaccid
- **Power:** weak
- **Reflexes:** absent and/or brisk
- **Sensory examination is normal**
- **Speech:** dysarthric, usually pseudo-bulbar ('hot potato' speech – UMN, due to a spastic tongue) or bulbar (nasal, 'Donald Duck' speech, LMN from flaccid tongue)
- **Tongue:** wasting and fasciculation (bulbar) or a stiff spastic tongue with brisk jaw jerk (pseudo-bulbar)
- Cognitive disturbance (accompanying frontotemporal dementia) when advanced
- No sensory, extra-ocular muscle, cerebellar or extra-pyramidal involvement

Discussion

- MND is a progressive disease of unknown aetiology
- There is axonal degeneration of upper and lower motor neurones
- Motor neurone disease may be classified into four types, although there is often some overlap:
  - ○ **Amyotrophic lateral sclerosis:** combined UMN and LMN signs
  - ○ **Primary lateral sclerosis:** only UMN signs
  - ○ **Progressive spinal muscular atrophy:** only LMN signs in limbs. *Best prognosis*
  - ○ **Progressive bulbar palsy:** only LMN signs in brainstem. *Worst prognosis*

INVESTIGATION

- Clinical diagnosis
- **EMG:** denervation
- **MRI (brain and c-spine):** to exclude cervical cord or brain-stem lesions (mimics)

TREATMENT

- Supportive, e.g. PEG feeding and NIPPV
- Multidisciplinary approach to care
- Riluzole (glutamate antagonist): slows disease progression by an average of 3 months but does not improve function or quality of life and is costly

PROGNOSIS

- Most die within 3 years of diagnosis from bronchopneumonia and respiratory failure. Some disease variants may survive longer
- Worst if elderly at onset, female and with bulbar involvement

Parkinson's disease

This man complains of slowness when walking/tremor. Examine him neurologically.

Clinical signs
- **Face:** Hypomimic with reduced spontaneous movements and blinking
- Coarse, pill-rolling, 3–5 Hz **tremor**
- **Bradykinesia:** ask to repeatedly oppose index finger onto thumb quickly; look for delay starting and movements getting slower and smaller
- **Cogwheel rigidity** at wrists (rigidity plus superimposed tremor)
- **Gait** is shuffling and festinant. Reduced arm swinging. Walking brings out tremor
- **Speech** is hypophonic and monotonous
- **In addition:**
  - ○ **Lying–standing BP:** significant drops seen in late PD (and worsened with levodopa or dopamine agonists). If seen early suggests **multisystem atrophy (MSA):** Parkinsonism with postural hypotension; cerebellar and pyramidal variants
  - ○ **Vertical eye movements:** in **progressive supranuclear palsy** vertical saccades are slow (i.e. the examiner can follow the eyes moving up/down); later patients cannot look up
  - ○ **Cognitive impairment or hallucinations:**
    - ○ Precede (or within 1 year of) onset, diagnosis = **dementia with Lewy bodies**
    - ○ later = **Parkinson's disease dementia**
- Ask for a **medication** history

Discussion
CAUSES OF PARKINSONISM
- Parkinson's disease (most common cause) – *asymmetrical*
- Parkinson-plus syndromes:
  - ○ Multisystem atrophy (autonomic failure) – *symmetrical*
  - ○ Progressive supranuclear palsy – *symmetrical*
  - ○ Corticobasal degeneration; unilateral Parkinsonian signs – *asymmetrical*
- Drug-induced, particularly prochlorperazine, metoclopramide, antipsychotics
- Vascular (acute basal ganglia stroke or diffuse small vessel disease)
- Post-encephalitis

PATHOLOGY
- Degeneration of the dopaminergic neurones between the substantia nigra and basal ganglia

TREATMENT
- **L-Dopa** with a peripheral dopa-decarboxylase inhibitor, e.g. co-beneldopa (Madopar®)
  - ○ Initially causes nausea (use domperidone – does not cross blood–brain barrier)
  - ○ Later can experience wearing off – addressed by more frequent dosing, modified-release preparations or addition of drug to reduce dopamine breakdown – COMT inhibitor (entacapone) or MAO inhibitor (selegiline) – and peak-dose dyskinesias (choreiform movements)
- **Dopamine agonists**, e.g. ropinirole: sometimes used in younger patients; slightly less effective and higher risk of impulsivity
- **Advanced therapies:** deep-brain stimulation or the dopamine agonist apomorphine (infusions or rescue injections)

CAUSES OF TREMOR

- Examine at rest (for Parkinsonism); then with arms outstretched (for postural); then during finger–nose testing (for kinetic)
- **Resting tremor:** (Parkinsonism – if asymmetrical usually Parkinson's disease)
- **Action tremor:**
  - **Postural tremor** (worse with arms outstretched):
    - Benign essential tremor (symmetrical, strong FH, better with EtOH)
    - Dystonic tremor (asymmetrical, coarser, changes with position; may have other features of dystonia, e.g. writer's cramp)
    - Enhanced physiological (anxiety, caffeine, hyperthyroid, EtOH withdrawal)
  - **Kinetic (intention tremor):** worsens towards point of intention (touching your finger)
    - Ipsilateral cerebellar lesion

Hereditary motor sensory neuropathy
aka Charcot–Marie–Tooth

This man complains of progressive weakness and a change in the appearance of his legs. Please examine him neurologically.

Clinical signs
- Wasting of distal lower limb muscles with preservation of the thigh muscle bulk (inverted champagne bottle appearance) and hand muscles
- Pes cavus (also in Friedreich's ataxia): indicates motor neuropathy during development
- Weakness of distal muscles, e.g. ankle dorsi-flexion, toe extension, fingers
- Distal (glove and stocking) sensory loss (usually mild)
- Gait is high stepping (due to foot drop)
- Palpable lateral popliteal nerve in most common subtype (1A)

Discussion
- Subtypes are divided according to neurophysiological findings (axonal vs demyelinating) and the inheritance pattern
- Type 1A (autosomal dominant demyelinating) is most common and is due to 17p duplication (contains *PMP22* gene)

Friedreich's ataxia
Examine this young man's neurological system.

Clinical signs
- Young adult, wheelchair (or ataxic gait)
- Pes cavus (also seen in HMSN)
- Bilateral cerebellar signs (see Cerebellar Syndrome)
- Combined UMN and LMN signs (e.g. leg wasting with absent reflexes due to the accompanying peripheral neuropathy with bilateral upgoing plantars due to corticospinal tract degeneration)
- Posterior column signs (loss of vibration and joint position sense)

Other signs
- Kyphoscoliosis
- Optic atrophy (30%)
- High-arched palate
- Sensorineural deafness (10%)
- Listen for murmur of HOCM
- Ask to dip urine (10% develop diabetes)

Discussion
- Inheritance is usually autosomal recessive
- Onset is during teenage years
- Survival rarely exceeds 20 years from diagnosis
- There is an association with HOCM and a mild dementia

Facial weakness

Examine this patient's cranial nerves. What is wrong?

Clinical signs
- Unilateral facial droop, reduced or absent nasolabial fold and forehead creases
- Inability to raise the eyebrows (frontalis), screw the eyes up (orbicularis oculi) or smile (orbicularis oris)
- Also examine V–VIIIth nerves and coordination (and limbs if time)

Level of the lesion and causes

Hemisphere MS, stroke, tumour	UMN	± Ipsilateral UMN features in limbs
Pons MS, stroke, tumour	UMN	± Ipsilateral UMN features in limbs ± Ipsilateral VI nerve palsy (as VII loops around VI in pons so lesions damage both)
Cerebellar-pontine angle Tumour, e.g. acoustic neuroma	LMN	+ V, VI, VIII and cerebellar signs (± scar behind ear)
Remaining course Cholesteatoma and abscess Ramsay Hunt syndrome (herpes zoster) Bell's palsy (see later)	LMN	+ VIII ± facial swelling + Painful vesicles in inner ear or tongue

DISTINGUISH UMN FROM LMN FACIAL WEAKNESS
- There is bilateral innervation of frontalis (forehead) and orbicularis oculi (eye closure):
  - UMN facial weakness **spares** the forehead and eye closure
  - LMN facial weakness **involves** the forehead and eye closure
  - **Bell's phenomenon:** eyeball normally rolls upwards on attempted eye closure (visible if orbicularis oculi weakness)

Discussion
COMMONEST CAUSE IS BELL'S PALSY
- Rapid onset (1–2 days)
- HSV-1 has been implicated
- Induced swelling and compression of the nerve within the facial canal causes demyelination and temporary conduction block
- Treatment: prednisolone commenced within 72 h of onset improves outcomes, plus aciclovir if severe
- **Remember eye protection** (artificial tears, tape eye closed at night)

- Prognosis: 70–80% make a full recovery
- Pregnancy: Bell's palsy is more common in pregnancy, and outcome may be worse

CAUSES OF BILATERAL LMN FACIAL WEAKNESS
- GBS (AIDP)
- Rarer causes: sarcoidosis, myasthenia gravis, Lyme disease, syphilis

Myasthenia gravis
Examine this patient's cranial nerves. She has been suffering with double vision.

Clinical signs
- Bilateral ptosis (worse on sustained upward gaze)
- Complicated bilateral extra-ocular muscle palsies
- Myasthenic snarl (on attempting to smile)
- Nasal speech, palatal weakness and poor swallow (bulbar involvement)
- Demonstrate proximal muscle weakness; if none look for proximal **fatiguability**
- Look for sternotomy scars (thymectomy)
- State that you would like to assess respiratory muscle function (FVC)

Discussion
- **Associations:** other autoimmune diseases, e.g. diabetes mellitus, rheumatoid arthritis, thyrotoxicosis, SLE and thymomas
- **Cause:** Anti-nicotinic acetylcholine receptor (anti-AChR) or anti-muscle-specific-kinase (MuSK) antibodies affect motor end-plate neurotransmission

INVESTIGATIONS
- **Diagnostic tests**
  - Anti-AChR antibodies positive in 80% of cases
  - Anti-MuSK antibodies often positive if anti-AChR negative
  - EMG: decrement of compound muscle action potential amplitude with repetitive stimulation
- **Other tests**
  - CT or MRI of the mediastinum (thymoma in 10%)
  - TFTs (Grave's present in 5%)
  - Send TPMT (enzyme metabolising azathioprine) if likely to need immunosuppression

TREATMENTS
- If purely ocular only need acetylcholinesterase inhibitor (e.g. pyridostigmine)
- Otherwise, need pyridostigmine plus immunosuppression:
  - Steroids (titrate up then wean down once stable; if deteriorate on withdrawal then need long-term steroid-sparing agent – azathioprine or mycophenolate)
- If bulbar or severe limb weakness consider IV immunoglobulin or plasma exchange
- Thymectomy in some subgroups (elective, not acute)

Lambert–Eaton myasthenic syndrome (LEMS)
- Pelvic then pectoral weakness plus autonomic (dry mouth and sphincter) with ptosis later
- Diminished reflexes that become brisker after exercise
- 70% paraneoplastic, especially small cell lung cancer
- Antibodies block pre-synaptic calcium channels
- **Investigations:**
  - Voltage-gated calcium channel antibodies
  - EMG: increment on repetitive stimulation
- **Treatment:**
  - Treat cause (immunosuppress if no cancer)
  - Potentiate synaptic transmission with 3,4-diaminopyridine for symptom control

Tuberous sclerosis

This patient has had a first seizure recently. Please examine them as you wish. What is the diagnosis?

Clinical signs

SKIN CHANGES

- Facial (perinasal: butterfly distribution) adenoma sebaceum (angiofibromata)
- Periungual fibromas (hands and feet)
- Shagreen patch: roughened, leathery skin over the lumbar region
- Ash leaf macules: depigmented macules on trunk (fluoresce with UV/Wood's light)

RESPIRATORY

- Cystic lung disease

ABDOMINAL

- Renal enlargement caused by polycystic kidneys and/or renal angiomyolipomata
- Transplanted kidney
- Signs of renal replacement therapy, e.g. dialysis fistulae

EYES

- Retinal phakomas (dense white patches) in 50%

CNS

- Learning difficulties may occur
- Seizures and signs of anti-epileptic use, e.g. phenytoin; gum hypertrophy

Discussion

- Autosomal dominant (*TSC1* on chromosome 9, *TSC2* on chromosome 16) with variable penetrance
- 80% have epilepsy (majority present in childhood, but adult presentation also seen)
- Cognitive defects in 50%

RENAL MANIFESTATIONS

- Include renal angiomyolipomas, renal cysts and renal cell carcinoma
- The genes for tuberous sclerosis and ADPKD are contiguous on chromosome 16, hence some mutations lead to both conditions
- Renal failure may result from cystic disease, or parenchymal destruction by massive angiomyolipomas

INVESTIGATION

- Skull films: 'railroad track' calcification
- CT/MRI head: tuberous masses in cerebral cortex (often calcify)
- Echo and abdominal ultrasound: hamartomas and renal cysts
- Previously known as **EPILOIA** (**EPI**lepsy, **LO**w **I**ntelligence, **A**denoma sebaceum)

Neurofibromatosis
Examine this patient's skin.

Clinical signs
- Cutaneous neurofibromas: two or more
- Café-au-lait patches: six or more, >15 mm diameter in adults
- Axillary freckling
- Lisch nodules: melanocytic hamartomas of the iris
- Blood pressure: hypertension (associated with renal artery stenosis and phaeochromocytoma)
- Examine the chest: fine crackles (honeycomb lung and fibrosis)
- Neuropathy with enlarged palpable nerves
- Visual acuity: optic glioma/compression

Discussion
- Inheritance is autosomal dominant
- Type I (chromosome 17) is the classical peripheral form
- Type II (chromosome 22) is central and presents with bilateral acoustic neuromas and sensi-neural deafness rather than skin lesions

ASSOCIATIONS
- Phaeochromocytoma (2%)
- Renal artery stenosis (2%)

COMPLICATIONS
- Epilepsy
- Sarcomatous change (5%)
- Scoliosis (5%)
- Mental retardation (10%)

CAUSES OF ENLARGED NERVES AND PERIPHERAL NEUROPATHY
- **Neurofibromatosis**
- HMSN (CMT1A subtype)
- Leprosy
- Amyloidosis
- Acromegaly
- Refsum's disease

Abnormal pupils
Examine this patient's eyes.

Horner's pupil

Clinical signs
- 'PEAS'

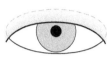
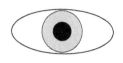

Horner's

Ptosis (levator palpebrae is partially supplied by sympathetic fibres);
Enophthalmos (sunken eye);
Anhydrosis (sympathetic fibres control sweating);
Small pupil (miosis).
May also have flushed/warm skin ipsilaterally to the Horner's pupil due to loss of vasomotor sympathetic tone to the face.

Other signs
- Look at the ipsilateral side of the neck for scars (trauma, e.g. central lines, carotid endarterectomy surgery or aneurysms) and tumours (Pancoast's)

Discussion
CAUSE
- **Following the sympathetic tract's anatomical course:**

Brain stem	Spinal cord	Neck
MS	Syrinx	Aneurysm
Stroke (Wallenberg's)		Trauma
		Pancoast's tumour (lung apex)

Holmes–Adie (myotonic) pupil

Clinical signs

Holmes–Adie pupil

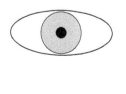
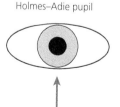

Moderately dilated pupil that has a poor response to light and a sluggish response to accommodation (you may have to wait!)

Light source

Other signs
• Absent or diminished ankle and knee jerks

Discussion
• A benign condition that is more common in females. Reassure the patient that nothing is wrong

Argyll Robertson pupil

Clinical signs

A–R pupil

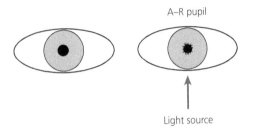

Small irregular pupil. Accommodates but doesn't react to light. Atrophied and depigmented iris.

Light source

Other signs
• Offer to look for sensory ataxia (tabes dorsalis):
  ○ **D**orsal column degeneration
  ○ **O**rthopaedic pain (Charcot joints)
  ○ **R**eflexes decreased
  ○ **S**hooting pain
  ○ **A**rgyll Robertson pupils
  ○ **L**ocomotor ataxia
  ○ **I**mpaired proprioception
  ○ **S**yphilis

Discussion
• Usually a manifestation of quaternary syphilis, but it may also be caused by diabetes mellitus
• Test for quaternary syphilis using TPHA or FTA, which remain positive for the duration of the illness
• Treat with penicillin

Oculomotor (III) nerve palsy

Clinical signs

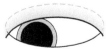

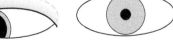

Ptosis usually complete. Dilated pupil. The eye points 'down and out' due to the unopposed action of lateral rectus (VI) and superior oblique (IV).

III nerve palsy

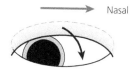

Nasal

Test for the trochlear (IV) nerve: on looking nasally the eye will intort (rotate towards the nose), indicating that the trochlear nerve is working.

- If the pupil is normal, consider medical causes of III palsy
- Surgical causes often impinge on the superficially located papillary fibres running in the III nerve

Discussion
CAUSES

Medical	Surgical
Mononeuritis multiplex, e.g. diabetes	**C**ommunicating artery aneurysm (posterior)
Midbrain infarction: Weber's	**C**avernous sinus pathology: thrombosis, tumour or fistula (IV, V and VI may also be affected)
Midbrain demyelination (MS)	
Migraine	**C**erebral uncus herniation

Optic atrophy

Clinical signs
- Relative afferent pupillary defect (RAPD)

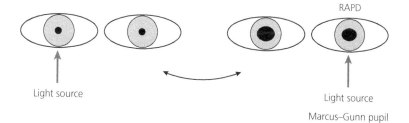

RAPD

Light source

Light source

Marcus–Gunn pupil

Dilatation of the pupil on moving the light source from the normal eye (consensual reflex) to the abnormal eye (direct reflex).

- Fundoscopy: disc pallor and possible causes

CAUSES:
ON EXAMINING THE FUNDUS
- **Glaucoma** (cupping of the disc)
- **Retinitis pigmentosa**
- **Central retinal artery occlusion**

- **Frontal brain tumour: Foster–Kennedy syndrome** (papilloedema in one eye due to raised intercranial pressure and optic atrophy in the other due to direct compression by the tumour)

AT A GLANCE FROM THE END OF THE BED
- Cerebellar signs, e.g. nystagmus: **MS** (internuclear ophthalmoplegia), **Friedreich's ataxia** (scoliosis and pes cavus)
- Large, bossed skull: **Paget's disease** (hearing aid)
- Argyll–Robertson pupil: **tertiary syphilis**

Discussion
CAUSES: 'PALE DISCS'
- **P**RESSURE*: tumour, glaucoma and Paget's
- **A**TAXIA: Friedreich's ataxia
- **LE**BER'S
- **D**IETARY: ↓B$_{12}$, **D**EGENERATIVE: retinitis pigmentosa
- **I**SCHAEMIA: central retinal artery occlusion
- **S**YPHILIS and other infections, e.g. CMV and toxoplasmosis
- **C**YANIDE and other toxins, e.g. alcohol, lead and tobacco
- **S**CLEROSIS: MS*
* denotes commonest cause

RETINAL PATHOLOGY

These cases may appear in isolation as part of the Neurology station, or within Consultations (e.g. retinal artery occlusion and AF). Other retinal pathology is covered elsewhere (e.g. diabetic and hypertensive retinopathy in Consultations).

Age-related macular degeneration

Examine this elderly patient's fundi. She complains of recent loss of vision.

Clinical signs

- Wet (neovascular and exudative) or dry (non-neovascular, atrophic and non-exudative)
- Macular changes:
  - Drusen (extracellular material)
  - Geographic atrophy
  - Fibrosis
  - Neovascularization (wet)

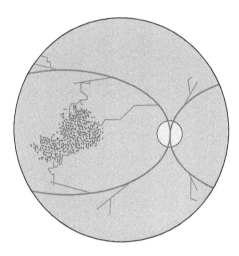

Multiple drusen (small yellowish deposits) around the macula – consistent with dry AMD; if neovascularization also present it is termed wet AMD.

Discussion

RISK FACTORS

- Age, white race, family history and smoking
- Wet AMD has a higher incidence of coronary heart disease and stroke

TREATMENT

- Ophthalmology referral
- Progression of wet AMD may be delayed by intravitreal injections of anti-VEGF (theoretically may increase cerebrovascular and cardiovascular risk)

PROGNOSIS

- Majority of patients with wet AMD progress to blindness in the affected eye within 2 years of diagnosis without treatment
- Dry AMD progresses much more slowly and many patients retain good vision until atrophic changes occur in the central foveal area

Retinitis pigmentosa

This man has been complaining of difficulty seeing at night. Please examine his eyes.

Clinical signs
- White stick and braille book (registered blind)
- Reduced peripheral field of vision (tunnel vision)
- Fundoscopy

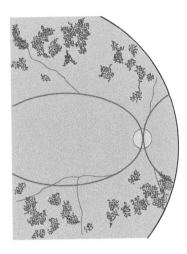

Peripheral retina 'bone spicule pigmentation', which follows the veins and spares the macula. Optic atrophy due to neuronal loss (consecutive). Association: cataract (absent red reflex).

AT A GLANCE FROM THE END OF THE BED
- **Ataxic:** Friedreich's ataxia, abetalipoproteinaemia, Refsum's disease, Kearns–Sayre syndrome
- **Deafness (hearing aid/white stick with red stripes):** Refsum's disease, Kearns–Sayre syndrome, Usher's disease
- **Ophthalmoplegia/ptosis and permanent pacemaker:** Kearns–Sayre syndrome
- **Polydactyly:** Laurence–Moon–Biedl syndrome
- **Ichthyosis:** Refsum's disease

Discussion
- Inherited form of retinal degeneration characterized by loss of photo receptors

CAUSES
- Congenital: often autosomal recessive inheritance, 15% due to rhodopsin pigment mutations
- Acquired: post-inflammatory retinitis

PROGNOSIS
- Progressive loss of vision due to retinal degeneration. Begins with reduced night vision. Most are registered blind at 40 years, with central visual loss in the seventh decade
- No treatment, although vitamin A may slow disease progression

Retinal artery occlusion
Examine this man's fundi.

Clinical signs (in acute phase)
- Pale, milky fundus with thread-like arterioles
- ± Cherry red macula (choroidal blood supply)
- **Cause:** AF (irregular pulse) or carotid stenosis (bruit)
- **Effect:** retinal and optic atrophy (chronic) and blindness in affected eye (white stick if both eyes affected)
- Note that branch retinal artery occlusion will have a field defect opposite to the quadrant of affected retina

Discussion
CAUSES
- **Embolic:** carotid plaque rupture or cardiac mural thrombus. Treatment: aspirin, anti-coagulation and endarterectomy
- **Giant cell arteritis:** tender scalp and pulseless temporal arteries. Treatment: empirical high-dose steroid urgently, check ESR and arrange temporal artery biopsy to confirm diagnosis

Retinal vein occlusion
Examine this patient's fundi.

Clinical signs
- Flame haemorrhages +++ radiating out from a swollen disc
- Engorged tortuous veins
- Cotton-wool spots
- **Cause:** look for diabetic or hypertensive changes (visible in branch retinal vein occlusion)
- **Effect:** Rubeosis iridis causes secondary glaucoma (in central retinal vein occlusion), visual loss or field defect

Discussion
CAUSES
- **Hypertension**
- **Hyperglycaemia:** diabetes mellitus
- **Hyperviscocity:** Waldenström's macroglobulinaemia or myeloma
- **High intraocular pressure:** glaucoma

Abdominal

Clinical mark sheet

Clinical skill	Satisfactory	Unsatisfactory
Physical examination	Correct, thorough, fluent, systematic, professional	Incorrect technique, omits, unsystematic, hesitant
Identifying physical signs	Identifies correct signs Does not find signs that are not present	Misses important signs Finds signs that are not present
Differential diagnosis	Constructs sensible differential diagnosis	Poor differential, fails to consider the correct diagnosis
Clinical judgement	Sensible and appropriate management plan	Inappropriate management Unfamiliar with management
Maintaining patient welfare	Respectful, sensitive Ensures comfort, safety and dignity	Causes physical or emotional discomfort Jeopardizes patient safety

Cases for PACES, Fourth Edition. Stephen Hoole, Andrew Fry and Rachel Davies.
© 2025 John Wiley & Sons Ltd. Published 2025 by John Wiley & Sons Ltd.

Abdominal exam – general advice

- Expose the patient's abdomen and lower chest – 'nipples to knees' is usually recommended, but remember to maintain the patient's modesty. Lie the patient flat
- What clues are you expecting to see from the end of the bed?
  - General body habitus – cachexia, ascites, abdominal masses. Cushingoid features, abnormal pigmentation
  - Jaundice
  - Abdominal scars
  - Arms – arteriovenous fistulae
  - Tunnelled dialysis lines (upper chest)
- Ask the patient to hold their hands up in front of them:
  - Tremor – tacrolimus
  - Nail signs – clubbing, koilonychia, etc.
  - Get them to cock their wrists – asterixis ('liver flap') – press gently back with your palm against their fingers and feel it if you're not sure
  - Wrist – take the pulse and look for arteriovenous fistulae
- As you move up the arm, always state that you would like to measure the blood pressure at this point
- Examine the face, looking for:
  - Sclera – jaundice
  - Conjunctival pallor (pull down one eyelid with your little finger)
  - Signs of other systemic disease with gastrointestinal pathology – scleroderma (beaked nose, small mouth with peri-oral furrowing), iron-deficiency anaemia (angular stomatitis), hereditary haemorrhagic telangiectasia (facial/oral telangiectasia)
  - Tongue, gums (hypertrophy) and dentition
- State that you would like to place the patient at 45° to examine the JVP, but try not to waste time actually doing this!
- Examine for cervical lymphadenopathy – you should be able to do this with equal proficiency from the front or back; only sit the patient up if they are able
- Move down the chest, looking in the axillae (loss of body hair, acanthosis nigricans, freckling), for gynaecomastia in men, current tunnelled dialysis catheters, Hickman lines (smaller diameter, usually single lumen) or portacaths (or scars from previous)
- Now you finally reach the abdomen – have another look for scars you may have missed earlier
- When you examine their abdomen, the following are key:
  - Ideally kneel down at an angle to the bed so that you are facing towards the head of the bed and the patient's face. You are going to examine with your right hand (to start with), but don't look directly at it. Peripheral vision is a wonderful thing
  - Keep your eyes on their face the whole time – you have to be alert for any discomfort you are causing
  - Gently feel around the abdomen with one hand in a systematic fashion. All you are doing at this point is assessing for peritonism – is there any rigidity or guarding, does the patient feel any pain? If the patient looks in discomfort, check with them that it is OK to proceed
  - Then feel for deeper masses, usually with two hands, one on top of the other, dipping down with your extended fingers by flexing at the MCPJs
  - If you feel a mass, characterize it – and don't move on until you have. You should be able to state where it is, approximate size, consistency, edge (smooth/irregular), if it is pulsatile, movement with respiration, and you might auscultate it and see if it trans-illuminates. Ideally this will give you an idea what it is
- Then palpate each organ in turn:
  - Liver – starting from the right iliac fossa, asking the patient to take deep breaths and feel for the liver edge with your hand steady in inspiration

- o Spleen – again starting from the right iliac fossa with your right hand (it helps to put your left hand behind the patient over their lowest left-sided ribs and pull upwards slightly), palpating with each inspiration up towards the left upper quadrant. If you're not sure, rolling the patient towards you, onto their right side (keeping your left hand behind their ribs t guide/support them) helps tip the spleen medially and may assist you
  - o Ballot each kidney
  - o Palpate for an abdominal aortic aneurysm
- Percuss the abdomen and look for ascites – start at the umbilicus and percuss towards the opposite flank. When you encounter dullness, keep your finger there and ask the patient to roll towards you. Wait 10 seconds and percuss again – if there is ascites what was dull should now be resonant. You can check by percussing back to the umbilicus – this should have been resonant and will now be dull (if ascites is present). This is shifting dullness
- Auscultate – over any mass, over hepatomegaly and centrally (bowel sounds)
- Feel femoral pulses and assess for lymphadenopathy. Also examine the legs for oedema – and see how high it extends
- Turn around to face the examiners and state that you would also like to do some of the following to complete your examination:
  - o Examine the external genitalia and hernial orifices
  - o Perform a rectal examination
  - o Perform urinalysis
  - o Check the blood pressure (if you forgot earlier)

Chronic liver disease and hepatomegaly

This man complains of weight loss and abdominal discomfort. His GP has referred him to you for a further opinion. Please examine his abdomen.

Clinical signs

SIGNS OF CHRONIC LIVER DISEASE

- **General:** cachexia, icterus (also in acute), excoriation and bruising
- **Hands:** leuconychia, clubbing, Dupuytren's contractures and palmar erythema
- **Face:** xanthelasma, parotid swelling and fetor hepaticus
- **Chest and abdomen:** spider naevi and caput medusa, reduced body hair, gynaecomastia and testicular atrophy (in males)

SIGNS OF HEPATOMEGALY

- Palpation and percussion:
    - Mass in the right upper quadrant that moves with respiration, that you are not able to get above and that is dull to percussion
    - Estimate size (finger breadths below the diaphragm)
    - Smooth or craggy/nodular (malignancy/cirrhosis)
    - Pulsatile (TR in CCF)
- Auscultation:
    - Bruit over liver (hepatocellular carcinoma)

EVIDENCE OF AN UNDERLYING CAUSE OF HEPATOMEGALY

- Tattoos and needle marks – infectious hepatitis
- Slate-grey pigmentation – haemochromatosis
- Cachexia – malignancy
- Mid-line sternotomy scar – CCF

EVIDENCE OF TREATMENT

- Ascitic drain/tap sites
- Surgical scars

EVIDENCE OF DECOMPENSATION

- **A**scites: shifting dullness
- **A**sterixis: 'liver flap'
- **A**ltered consciousness: encephalopathy

Discussion

CAUSES OF HEPATOMEGALY

- The **big three:**
    - **Cirrhosis** (alcoholic)
    - **Carcinoma** (metastases to liver)
    - **Congestive cardiac failure**
- Plus:
    - **I**nfectious (HBV and HCV)
    - **I**mmune (PBC, PSC and AIH)
    - **I**nfiltrative (amyloid and myeloproliferative disorders)

INVESTIGATIONS

- Bloods: FBC, clotting, U&E, LFT and glucose
- Ultrasound scan of abdomen
- Tap ascites (if present)

- Liver screen bloods:
  - Autoantibodies and immunoglobulins (PBC, PSC and AIH)
  - Hepatitis B and C serology
  - Ferritin (haemochromatosis)
  - Caeruloplasmin (Wilson's disease)
  - α-1 antitrypsin
  - AFP (hepatocellular carcinoma)
- Hepatic synthetic function: INR (acute) and albumin (chronic)
- Liver biopsy (diagnosis and staging)
- ERCP/MRCP (diagnose/exclude PSC)

IF MALIGNANCY
- Imaging: CXR and CT chest/abdomen/pelvis
- Colonoscopy/gastroscopy
- Biopsy (of liver lesion)

COMPLICATIONS OF CIRRHOSIS
- Variceal haemorrhage due to portal hypertension
- Hepatic encephalopathy
- Spontaneous bacterial peritonitis

CHILD–PUGH CLASSIFICATION OF CIRRHOSIS
Prognostic score based on bilirubin/albumin/INR/ascites/encephalopathy

	Score	1 year survival (%)
A	5–6	100
B	7–9	81
C	10–15	45

CAUSES OF ASCITES
- **C**irrhosis (80%)
- **C**arcinomatosis
- **C**CF

TREATMENT OF ASCITES IN CIRRHOTICS
- Abstinence from alcohol
- Salt restriction
- Diuretics (aim 1 kg weight loss/day)
- Liver transplantation

CAUSES OF PALMAR ERYTHEMA
- Cirrhosis
- Hyperthyroidism
- Rheumatoid arthritis
- Pregnancy
- Polycythaemia

- Physiological: puberty and senility
- Kleinfelter's syndrome
- Cirrhosis
- Drugs, e.g. spironolactone and digoxin
- Testicular tumour/orchidectomy
- Endocrinopathy, e.g. hyper-/hypothyroidism and Addison's

AUTOANTIBODIES IN LIVER DISEASE
- Primary biliary cirrhosis (PBC): antimitochondrial antibody (M2 subtype) in 98%, increased IgM
- Primary sclerosing cholangitis (PSC): ANA, anti-smooth muscle may be positive
- Autoimmune hepatitis (AIH): anti-smooth muscle, anti-liver/kidney microsomal type 1 (LKM1) and occasionally ANA may be positive (pattern helps classify)

Haemochromatosis

This 52 year-old man was referred after a diagnosis of diabetes mellitus was made by his GP. Please examine him and discuss further investigations.

Clinical signs
- Increased skin pigmentation (slate-grey colour)
- Stigmata of chronic liver disease
- Hepatomegaly

SCARS
- Venesection
- Liver biopsy
- Joint replacement
- Abdominal rooftop incision (hemihepatectomy for hepatocellular carcinoma)

EVIDENCE OF COMPLICATIONS
- **Endocrine:** 'bronze diabetes' (e.g. injection sites), hypogonadism and testicular atrophy
- **Cardiac:** congestive cardiac failure
- **Joints:** arthropathy (pseudo-gout)

Discussion

INHERITANCE
- Autosomal recessive on chromosome 6
- *HFE* gene mutation: regulator of gut iron absorption
- Homozygous prevalence 1 : 300, carrier rate 1 : 10
- Males affected at an earlier age than females – protected by menstrual iron losses

PRESENTATION
- Fatigue and arthritis
- Chronic liver disease
- Incidental diagnosis or family screening

INVESTIGATION
- ↑ Serum ferritin
- ↑ Transferrin saturation
- Liver biopsy (diagnosis + staging)
- Genotyping
- And consider:
  - Blood glucose, HbA1c – diabetes
  - ECG, CXR, ECHO – cardiac failure
  - Liver ultrasound, α-fetoprotein – hepatocellular carcinoma (HCC)

TREATMENT
- Regular venesection (1 unit/week) until iron deficient, then venesect 1 unit 3–4 times/ year
- Avoid alcohol
- Surveillance for HCC

FAMILY SCREENING (1ST DEGREE RELATIVES AGED >20 YEARS)
- Iron studies (ferritin and TSAT)
- If positive:
  - Liver biopsy
  - Genotype analysis

PROGNOSIS
- 200× increased risk of HCC if cirrhotic
- Reduced life expectancy if cirrhotic
- Normal life expectancy without cirrhosis + effective treatment

Splenomegaly

This man presents with tiredness and lethargy. Please examine his abdominal system and discuss your diagnosis.

Clinical signs

GENERAL
- Anaemia
- Lymphadenopathy (axillae, cervical and inguinal areas)
- Purpura

ABDOMINAL
- Left upper quadrant mass that moves inferomedially with respiration, has a notch, is dull to percussion and you cannot get above nor ballot
- Estimate size
- Ensure that this is not an enlarged left kidney!
- Check for hepatomegaly

UNDERLYING CAUSE
- Lymphadenopathy – haematological and infective
- Anaemia, purpura – haematological
- Stigmata of chronic liver disease – cirrhosis with portal hypertension
- Splinter haemorrhages, murmur, etc. – bacterial endocarditis
- Rheumatoid hands – Felty's syndrome

Discussion

CAUSES
- Massive splenomegaly (>8 cm):
  - Myeloproliferative disorders (**CML** and **myelofibrosis**)
  - Tropical infections (**malaria**, visceral leishmaniasis, kala-azar)
- Moderate splenomegaly (4–8 cm):
  - Myelo-/lymphoproliferative disorders
  - Infiltration (Gaucher's and amyloidosis)
- Tip of spleen(<4 cm):
  - Myelo/lymphoproliferative disorders
  - Portal hypertension
  - Infections (EBV, infective endocarditis and infective hepatitis)
  - Haemolytic anaemia

INVESTIGATIONS
- Ultrasound abdomen
- **If haematological:**
  - FBC and film
  - CT chest and abdomen
  - Bone marrow aspirate and trephine
  - Lymph node biopsy
- **If infectious:**
  - Thick and thin films, antigen test (malaria)
  - Viral serology

INDICATIONS FOR SPLENECTOMY
- Rupture (trauma)
- Haematological (ITP and hereditary spherocytosis)

- Vaccination (ideally 2/52 prior to protect against encapsulated bacteria):
  - Pneumococcus
  - Meningococcus
  - *Haemophilus influenzae* (Hib)
- Prophylactic penicillin (lifelong)
- Medic alert bracelet

Distinguishing an enlarged left kidney from a spleen

	Spleen	Left kidney
Movement on respiration	Inferomedially (towards right iliac fossa)	Downwards and slightly laterally (in paracolic gutter)
Can you get above it?	No (arises from under ribcage)	Yes
Ballotable?	No	Yes
Percussion note?	Dull (nothing overlying)	Resonant (overlying small bowel)
Notch?	Yes	No

Renal enlargement

This woman has been referred by her GP for investigation of hypertension. Please examine her abdomen.

Clinical signs

PERIPHERAL
- Blood pressure: **hypertension**
- Arteriovenous fistulae (is it working? - thrill and bruit), tunnelled dialysis line (or scars from)
- Immunosuppressant 'stigmata', e.g. Cushingoid habitus due to steroids, gum hypertrophy with ciclosporin

ABDOMEN
- Palpable kidney: ballotable, can get above it and moves with respiration
- Polycystic kidneys: both may/should be palpable and can be grossly enlarged (will feel 'cystic' or nodular)
- Iliac fossae: scar with (or without if removed) transplanted kidney
- Ask to dip the urine: proteinuria and haematuria
- Ask to examine the external genitalia (varicocele in males)

ASSOCIATED CONDITIONS
- Hepatomegaly: polycystic kidney disease
- Indwelling urethral catheter: obstructive nephropathy with hydronephrosis
- Peritoneal dialysis catheter/scars

Discussion

CAUSES OF UNILATERAL ENLARGEMENT
- Polycystic kidney disease (other kidney not palpable or contralateral nephrectomy – flank scar)
- Renal cell carcinoma
- Simple cysts
- Hydronephrosis (due to ureteric obstruction)

CAUSES OF BILATERAL ENLARGEMENT
- Polycystic kidney disease
- Bilateral renal cell carcinoma (5%)
- Bilateral hydronephrosis
- Tuberous sclerosis (renal angiomyolipomata and cysts)
- Amyloidosis

INVESTIGATIONS
- U&E
- Urinalysis
- Urine cytology
- Ultrasound abdomen
- Renal biopsy if suspecting intrinsic renal disease
- CT if carcinoma is suspected
- Genetic studies (ADPKD)

Autosomal dominant polycystic kidney disease
- Progressive replacement of normal kidney tissue by cysts leading to renal enlargement and renal failure (5% of end-stage renal failure in UK)
- Prevalence 1 : 1000
- Genetics: 85% *ADPKD1* chromosome 16; 15% *ADPKD2* chromosome 4

- Presents with:
  - Hypertension
  - Recurrent UTIs
  - Abdominal pain (bleeding into cyst and cyst infection)
  - Abdominal/back pain – from massive renal enlargement
  - Macroscopic haematuria (bleeding into cysts)
  - Or as part of familial screening
- End-stage renal failure by age 40–60 years (earlier in *ADPKD1* than *-2*)
- Other organ involvement:
  - Hepatic cysts and hepatomegaly (rarely liver failure)
  - Intracranial Berry aneurysms (neurological sequelae/craniotomy scar?)
  - Mitral valve prolapse
- Genetic counselling of family and family screening; 10% represent new mutations
- Treatment: tolvaptan (vasopressin V2 receptor antagonist delays disease progression in those with moderate CKD), nephrectomy for recurrent bleeds/infection/size, dialysis and renal transplantation

The liver transplant patient
Please examine this man's abdomen.

Clinical signs
- Abdominal scars:

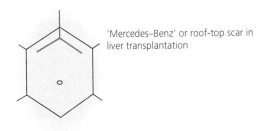

'Mercedes–Benz' or roof-top scar in liver transplantation

- Evidence of chronic liver disease

REASON FOR LIVER TRANSPLANTATION
- Slate-grey pigmentation – haemochromatosis
- Other autoimmune disease – PBC
- Tattoos and needle marks – hepatitis B, C

EVIDENCE OF IMMUNOSUPPRESSIVE MEDICATION
- Ciclosporin: gum hypertrophy and hypertension
- Steroids: Cushingoid appearance, thin skin, ecchymoses
- Tacrolimus: tremor

Discussion
TOP THREE REASONS FOR LIVER TRANSPLANTATION
- Cirrhosis
- Acute hepatic failure (hepatitis A and B, paracetamol overdose)
- Hepatic malignancy (hepatocellular carcinoma)

SUCCESS OF LIVER TRANSPLANTATION
- 90% 1-year survival
- 80% 5-year survival

CAUSES OF GUM HYPERTROPHY
- Drugs: ciclosporin, phenytoin and nifedipine
- Scurvy
- Acute myelomonocytic leukaemia
- Pregnancy
- Familial

SKIN SIGNS IN (ANY) TRANSPLANT PATIENTS
- **Malignancy**
  - Dysplastic change (actinic keratoses)
  - Squamous cell carcinoma (100× increased risk and multiple lesions)
  - Basal cell carcinoma and malignant melanoma (10× increased risk)
- **Infection:**
  - Viral warts
  - Cellulitis

The renal patient
Please examine this man's abdomen.

Clinical signs
- Stigmata:
  - Arms: arteriovenous fistula(e) – currently working (thrill), being used (thrill and dressings) or failed
  - Neck: tunnelled dialysis line (or previous lines; scars in the root of the neck and over the chest wall)
  - Abdominal scars:

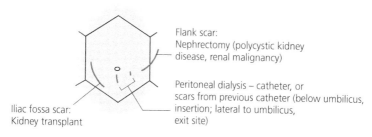

Flank scar:
Nephrectomy (polycystic kidney disease, renal malignancy)

Peritoneal dialysis – catheter, or scars from previous catheter (below umbilicus, insertion; lateral to umbilicus, exit site)

Iliac fossa scar:
Kidney transplant

- Fluid status (leg oedema)

THREE THINGS TO CONSIDER IN ALL RENAL PATIENTS
1. **Underlying reason for renal failure**
   - Polycystic kidneys: ADPKD
   - Visual impairment, fingerprick marks, injection sites/pump/CGM, etc. – diabetes
   - Sclerodactyly, typical facies – systemic sclerosis
   - Rheumatoid hands, nodules – rheumatoid arthritis
   - (Hepato)splenomegaly – amyloidosis
   - Other organ transplantation (liver/heart/lungs) – calcineurin inhibitor nephrotoxicity
   - Ungual fibromata, adenoma sebaceum, polycystic kidneys – tuberous sclerosis
2. **Current treatment modality**
   - Haemodialysis – working fistula, tunnelled neck lines, arteriovenous grafts
   - Peritoneal dialysis – abdominal catheter
   - Functioning transplant – no evidence of other current dialysis access (in use)
3. **Complications of past/current treatment**
   - Side effects of treatment for the underlying disease – Cushingoid appearance from steroids (glomerulonephritis)
   - Side effects of immunosuppressive treatment in transplant patients:
     - Fine tremor (tacrolimus)
     - Steroid side effects
     - Gum hypertrophy (ciclosporin)
     - Hypertension (ciclosporin, tacrolimus)
     - Significant leg oedema, mouth ulcers (sirolimus)
     - Skin damage and malignancy (especially ciclosporin and azathioprine)
   - Scars from previous access for dialysis, failed transplant(s)

KIDNEY–PANCREAS TRANSPLANTATION
- Consider if:
  - Lower midline abdominal incision, with a palpable kidney in an iliac fossa (but no overlying scar). The pancreas is intraperitoneal and not palpable

- ○ Evidence of previous diabetes (e.g. visual impairment)
- ○ Patient is younger (most commonly transplanted in 30s–40s)

Discussion

TOP THREE CAUSES FOR RENAL TRANSPLANTATION

- Glomerulonephritis
- Diabetic nephropathy
- Polycystic kidney disease (ADPKD)

PROBLEMS FOLLOWING TRANSPLANTATION

- **Rejection:** acute or chronic
- **Infection secondary to immunosuppression:**
  - ○ *Pneumocystis carinii*
  - ○ CMV
- **Increased risk of other pathology:**
  - ○ Skin malignancy
  - ○ Post-transplant lymphoproliferative disease
  - ○ Hypertension and hyperlipidaemia causing cardiovascular disease
- **Immunosuppressant drug side effects/toxicity:**
  - ○ Ciclosporin nephrotoxicity
- **Recurrence of original disease**
- **Chronic graft dysfunction**

SUCCESS OF RENAL TRANSPLANTATION

- 95% 1-year graft survival
- 50% 15-year graft survival (better with living-related donor grafts)

Communication

Clinical mark sheet

Clinical skill	Satisfactory	Unsatisfactory
Clinical communication skills	Relevant, accurate, clear, structured, comprehensive, fluent, professional	Omits important information Inaccurate, unclear, unstructured, uses jargon, unpractised, does not involve patient/relative in management plan
Managing patients' concerns	Seeks, detects and addresses concerns Actively listens, confirms understanding, empathetic	Overlooks concerns, poor listening, not empathetic Does not check patient understanding
Clinical judgement	Sensible and appropriate management plan, applies clinical/legal/ethical knowledge appropriately	Inappropriate management Does not apply clinical, legal or ethical knowledge to the case
Maintaining patient welfare	Respectful, sensitive Ensures comfort, safety and dignity	Causes physical or emotional discomfort Jeopardizes patient safety

Cases for PACES, Fourth Edition. Stephen Hoole, Andrew Fry and Rachel Davies.
© 2025 John Wiley & Sons Ltd. Published 2025 by John Wiley & Sons Ltd.

Communication station – general advice

- This station assesses the candidate's ability to hold a professional discussion with a patient or surrogate
  - The examiners are looking to ensure that all candidates are able to impart medical information in such a way that the patient can understand, that the candidate can assess and address the patient's concerns and, finally, that they can formulate, communicate and agree a management plan with the patient
  - Candidates will also be assessed on their understanding and application of ethics and medico-legal law in the UK
  - Familiarity with the GMC's Good Medical Practice (GMP) code is required to perform well in this station. While the main points of GMP are highlighted, where relevant, in the cases in this section, it is advisable to refresh your memory of this important document. It is the blueprint for ethical behaviour of all doctors within the UK
  - It is also key to understand a few key legal cases pertaining to medical practice. Again, these are covered in this section, but is imperative that you understand these points of law and are able to apply them to a variety of clinical scenarios
- Cases in this section fall into three broad categories: imparting medical information, breaking bad news and difficult ethical, legal or patient issues
  - While imparting medical information scenarios may seem intuitive and easy, these are often done poorly if lacking in a clear structure; this station is a key discriminator of a well or poorly prepared candidate.
  - The best preparation is to practise with a colleague acting as a surrogate patient to ensure that you make the most of the 10 minutes allocated and demonstrate that you possess all the clinical skills required to pass this station: communication, ability to manage and address the patient's concerns, clinical judgement, as well as always maintaining patient welfare
- In the new format PACES2023, this station has been split into two separate 10-minute stations that precede the respiratory and abdominal stations with no discussions with the examiners. You will therefore need to carefully read the question and plan your approach in the 5 minutes allotted before entering the examination room. You will not benefit from helpful prompts from examiners' questioning to demonstrate your knowledge; it is all down to your performance alone
  - A good tip is to note down headings of key discussion points that you must cover and also ensure that you are clear about the ethical or legal aspects of the case that you should raise
- Consider the clinical skills on the mark sheet that the examiners will be assessing. It is a professional interview, and the examiners will be watching to see if you address each of these specific areas. It is not enough to just be 'nice' to the patient in this station
- You will need to be able to demonstrate not only good communication but also that you are actively listening to the patient's concerns and addressing them with an appropriate plan.
  - Alongside this, you will need to demonstrate good clinical judgement while considering any ethical elements of the case and show the examiners that you are behaving in a non-judgmental and fair manner
  - Finally, you must ensure that the patient is always at the centre of any management plan and that you are mindful of any specific personal requirements that the patient has in order to ensure their welfare is prioritised
- During this station, there will be a bell 2 minutes before the end of the communication time. Please look out for this cue: it should prompt you to start to wrap up your discussion
  - The examiners will be looking to assess your ability to address any concerns that the patient has had. You will therefore need to use these 2 minutes to recap the plan and agree further actions with the patient prior to offering them any written information and agreeing when you will review them again

ETHICS AND LAW IN MEDICINE

Principles of medical ethics

- Most ethical dilemmas can be resolved, at least in part, by considering the four cornerstones of any ethical argument, namely **autonomy, beneficence, non-maleficence** and **justice**
  - **Autonomy** 'self-rule': respecting and following the patient's decisions in the management of their condition
  - **Beneficence:** promoting what is in the patient's best interests
  - **Non-maleficence:** avoiding harm
  - **Justice:** doing what is good for the population as a whole; distributing resources fairly
- There is often not a right or wrong answer to tricky ethical problems, but this framework enables informed discussion

EXAMPLE
- PEG feeding a semi-conscious patient post CVA:
  - **Autonomy:** the patient wishes to be fed or not
  - **Beneficence** and **non-maleficence:** feeding may improve nutritional status and aid recovery, but with risks of complication from the insertion of the PEG tube and subsequent aspiration. Also, the patient's poor quality of life may be lengthened
  - **Justice:** heavy resource burden looking after PEG-fed patients in nursing homes

Medico-legal system

- The legal system of England and Wales (the Scottish legal system is different) is defined by **common (case) law** and **statute law (Acts of Parliament)** and may be subdivided into **public (criminal) law** and **private (civil) law**
- Court decisions follow **judicial precedent** – they follow judgments that have gone before
- Medical malpractice is commonly a breach of the **law of tort** (part of civil law) and the most important aspects are **negligence** and **battery** (part of the tort of trespass)
- The judge must decide on the balance of probabilities (rather than beyond reasonable doubt – criminal law), whether the defendant(s) (doctor and hospital NHS Trust) are liable and whether the claimant is due compensation

Negligence

- This is the commonest reason for a doctor to go to court. Claimants need to prove:
  1. The doctor had a duty of care:
     - Doctors (unless they are GPs in their geographical practice) are not legally obliged to act as 'good Samaritans' (although morally they may be)
  2. There was a breach of the appropriate standard of care:
     - **Bolam test:** the doctor is not negligent if they acted in accordance with a responsible/reasonable/respectable body of medical opinion (even if that opinion is in the minority)
     - **Bolitho test:** the opinion must also withstand logical analysis
  3. The breach of the duty of care caused harm

Competency and consent

A competent patient

- *Every human being of adult years and of sound mind has a right to determine what shall be done to their own body*
- In accepting a patient's autonomy to determine the course of management, the clinician must be satisfied that the patient has capacity. If this is not the case, the doctor should act in the patient's best interests
- Consent is only valid when the individual has capacity (or in legal terms, 'is competent'):
  - A patient does not lack capacity just because they act against their best interests
  - Capacity is not a global term but is specific to each decision, i.e. a patient may be competent to make a will but at the same time incompetent to consent to treatment
  - A clinician does not have to prove beyond all reasonable doubt that a patient has capacity, only that the balance of probability favours capacity

Assessing capacity

- In order to be assessed as having capacity to make a specific decision, a patient must be able to:
  1. Comprehend and retain the information needed
  2. Understand the pros and cons of both accepting and refusing the proposed plan
  3. Be free from undue external influence
  4. Communicate their response
- Patients under 16 years of age can consent to accept and undergo treatment, but not to refuse treatment, if they are deemed '**Gillick competent**', i.e. are deemed mature enough to understand the implications of their actions. Refusal of consent to treatment may be overridden by a parent or a court, if it is in the child's best interest

Legal aspects

- **Assault** is a threat or an attempt to physically injure another person, whereas **battery** is actual (direct or indirect) physical contact or injury without consent. They are usually civil rather criminal offences
- **Implied consent:** if a patient goes to hospital and holds out their arm to allow a medical practitioner to take their pulse, written or verbal consent is not necessary
- **Consent documentation:** the legal basis for informed consent changed in 2015.
  - The **Montgomery v Lanarkshire** case challenged how much information a patient should receive about the risks of a procedure to ensure informed consent
  - The ruling stated that if there was a significant risk that could affect the decision made by a reasonable patient about their options, then it would be expected that a doctor would inform a patient of that risk
  - The ruling also makes it clear that any intervention must be based on a shared decision-making process, ensuring the patient is aware of all options and supported to make an informed choice by their healthcare professional
- The GMC's GMP guidelines suggest that you should try to ascertain what potential risks matter to the individual patient when you are consenting them. For example, by asking: 'Is there anything that you are worried about with regard to this procedure?'
- It is possible to not discuss a potential risk if you feel that the patient you are talking to would be overly distressed by that piece of information or they have requested not to know. However, this should be the exception to the rule rather than an option routinely taken
- In general, it is advisable to tell the patient of all potential serious complications and those with an incidence of at least 1%
- A signed consent form is not legally binding – patients may withdraw consent at any time. It is not illegal to operate without a consent form (as long as verbal or implied

consent has been obtained). However, it provides admissible evidence that consent has been obtained

- If the patient lacks capacity, it is best practice to discuss any intended procedure with a relative and for their agreement to be documented on the consent form, but this is not legally binding and does not constitute consent

The Mental Capacity Act (2005)

- The Mental Capacity Act (which is a separate Act to the Mental Health Act) was introduced to protect people who cannot make decisions for themselves. It enables people to appoint someone on their behalf in case they become unable to make decisions for themselves in the future
- There are three parts to this act that you need to be aware of:
  - **Appointment of a deputy:** an individual can nominate a deputy to make decisions with regard to monetary matters
    - An individual needs to be legally competent when this application is made and the application needs to be accepted by the Court of Protection to be valid
    - The deputy must make decisions in accordance with the best interests of the individual
    - A deputy does not have the right to make decisions about medical or welfare issues on behalf of the individual
  - **Appointment of a lasting power of attorney:** an attorney appointed through a lasting power of attorney application has two roles: first to act on behalf of an individual with regard to monetary and property matters, and also, in the event of a person losing capacity to make medical or welfare decisions, to act as a patient proxy; that is, the opinion of the attorney needs to be taken into account as if it were the opinion of the patient themselves
    - An application has to be signed by a solicitor and then registered with the Office of the Public Guardian. There is a separate form for each role and different individuals can be appointed for each task
    - The attorney must act in the best interests of the individual and abide by the Code of Practice
    - If anyone disputes the decision of an attorney, particularly if they are refusing life-saving treatment, the Court of Protection ultimately adjudicates on the decision
    - Just as with a patient, an attorney cannot demand treatment that is deemed to be clinically inappropriate
  - **Independent Mental Capacity Advocate:** when a person loses capacity and has not previously appointed a deputy or attorney, the Public Guardian, through the Court of Protection, can appoint an independent person to help with welfare and monetary decisions. They will liaise with doctors, nurses and social workers to agree a decision in the best interests of the patient

The Mental Health Act

- The **Mental Health Act 1983** can only be evoked to treat psychiatric illness in non-consenting patients
- **Section 5(2): emergency doctor's holding power:**
  - Applied by a physician of any specialty on an *in-patient* to enable a psychiatric assessment to be made
  - 72 hours' duration
  - Good practice to convert this to a Section 2 or 3
- **Section 2: admission for assessment order:**
  - Applied by two written medical recommendations (usually a psychiatrist and a GP) and an approved social worker or relative, on a patient *in the community*

- 28 days' duration
- May be converted to a Section 3
- The patient has a right of appeal to a tribunal within 14 days of detention
- **Section 3: admission for treatment order:**
  - Applied as in a Section 2 on a patient already diagnosed with a mental disorder
  - 6 months' duration then reviewed
- **Section 4: emergency admission to hospital order:**
  - Applied by one doctor (usually a GP) and an approved social worker or relative
  - Urgent necessity is demonstrable
  - May be converted to a Section 2 or 3

Confidentiality
- Confidentiality is an implied contract necessary for a successful doctor–patient relationship
- Without it, a patient's autonomy and privacy are compromised, trust is lost and the relationship weakened

GMC Guidelines
- *Confidentiality: Protecting and Providing Information*, **September 2000, Section 1 – Patients' right to confidentiality, Paragraph 1:**
  - 'Patients have the right to expect that doctors will not disclose any personal information which they learn during the course of their professional duties, unless the patient gives specific permission (preferably in writing). Without assurances about confidentiality patients may be reluctant to give doctors the information they need to provide good care.'

Legal aspects
- Patients usually complain to the GMC rather than sue if there has been a breach of confidentiality
- Under common law doctors are legally obliged to maintain confidentiality, although this obligation is not absolute
- Maintenance of confidentiality is a public not a private interest – it is in the public's interest to be able to trust a doctor. Therefore, breaching confidentiality is a question of balancing public interests
- Doctors have **discretion** to breach confidentiality when another party may be at serious risk of harm, e.g. an epileptic who continues to drive (the GMC advises doctors to inform the DVLA medical officer) or a patient who has HIV who refuses to tell their sexual partner. Doctors may also share information within the medical team
- Doctors **must** breach confidentiality to the relevant authorities in the following situations:
  - Notifiable diseases
  - Drug addiction
  - Abortion
  - In vitro fertilization
  - Organ transplant
  - Births and deaths
  - Police request
  - Search warrant signed by a circuit judge
  - Court order
  - Prevention, apprehension or prosecution of terrorists or perpetrators of serious crime

How to do it
- No breach of confidentiality has occurred if a patient gives consent, or the patient cannot be identified
- If consent is not given to disclose information but a physician deems that a breach in confidentiality is necessary, the patient should be notified in writing of the reason for disclosure, the content, to whom the disclosure has been made and the likely consequence for the patient
- The GMC provides guidelines on when confidentiality may be breached, which do not have the force of the law but are taken seriously by the courts. These guidelines may be consulted at www.gmc-uk.org

End-of-life decisions
- This is a contentious area and medical opinion is diverse

Sanctity of life
- The view that whenever possible human life should be maintained could be argued as ethically unjustified if extending that life results in suffering (non-maleficence) and if trivial life extension occurs at enormous monetary expense (justice)

Killing versus letting die
- In the former the doctor actively causes the patient's death; in the latter the patient's illness causes death, i.e. 'nature takes its course' while the doctor is passive
- Some people disagree, stating that the decisions to act or to omit to act are both 'active' choices, which may make it more difficult to morally justify

Withholding versus withdrawing treatment
- Although it may be easier to withhold treatment, rather than to withdraw that which has been started already, there are no legal or necessarily moral distinctions between the two
- Withdrawing treatment is considered in law to be a passive act and not killing

EXAMPLE
- A hospital trust was granted permission by the House of Lords to discontinue artificial hydration and nutrition in a young patient in a persistent vegetative state (*Airedale NHS Trust v Bland*, 1993)
- This case established the equivalence of withholding and withdrawing care and that the basic provisions of food and water are classified as medical treatments that could be withdrawn

Doctrine of double effect
- This is a moral argument that distinguishes actions that are intended to harm versus those where harm is foreseen but not intended

EXAMPLE
- The administration of morphine intended to palliate pain in a patient with a terminal illness may have the foreseen consequence of respiratory arrest and subsequent death
- It is morally and legally acceptable though, because the primary aim is to alleviate pain, not cause death

Do not attempt cardiopulmonary resuscitation (DNA-CPR) orders
- In 2014, a case was brought to the UK Court of Appeal (*Tracey v Cambridgeshire NHS Foundation Hospitals Trust*) by a family questioning whether or not it was against Article 8 of the Human Rights Act not to discuss DNA-CPR orders with a patient or their family
- The judge ruled in favour of Tracey and it is therefore now a legal obligation for medical staff to consult a patient or, in the situation where a patient lacks capacity, their family or advocate, when a decision to withhold potentially life-saving treatment is being considered, including DNA-CPR
- Failure to discuss these decisions could potentially result in legal action and it is no longer acceptable to avoid these discussions on the grounds that they may cause undue distress to the patient or family
- The ReSPECT (Recommended Summary Plan for Emergency Care and Treatment) process creates a summary of advanced personalized recommendations for a person's clinical care in a future emergency, e.g. cardiac arrest, when they will not have capacity

to make or express a choice. The process facilitates discussion and respects both patient preferences and clinical judgement. The agreed realistic clinical recommendations may be recorded on a ReSPECT form

- It is important to realize that this ruling does not state that CPR must be offered to all patients; it is merely stating that the decision whether or not to perform CPR must be discussed with the patient. English law still states that doctors are not required to administer futile treatment, and this can include CPR

Euthanasia

- Euthanasia is intentional killing, i.e. murder under English law, and is therefore illegal
- Assisted suicide, i.e. helping someone take their own life, is also a criminal offence

ARGUMENTS FOR

- Respecting a patient's autonomy over their body
- Beneficence, i.e. 'mercy killing', may prevent suffering
- Suicide is legal but is unavailable to the disabled

ARGUMENTS AGAINST

- Good palliative care obviates the need for euthanasia
- Risk of manipulation/coercion/exploitation of the vulnerable
- Undesirable practices will occur when constraints on killing are loosened (**'slippery-slope' argument**)

TYPES OF COMMUNICATION

Information delivery
- Communication skills are frequently assessed by the candidate's ability to inform the patient about their medical condition. These scenarios are often executed poorly by candidates in the PACES examination
- Make sure that you conduct a structured interview and that you have time to cover all relevant points
- Candidates often underestimate how difficult it is to do these scenarios well. Think about what you might say in a given scenario in advance of the exam

Approach to the discussion
- Introduce yourself and establish the reason for the discussion
- Assess the patient's level of knowledge:
  - First, discuss the nature of the condition that they have been diagnosed with
  - Give the information in simple language, avoiding medical jargon
  - Rehearse prior to the examination a description of all common medical complaints
- Facilitate questions and answer them, but avoid digressing too much
- Next discuss the medication they are going home on:
  - Make sure that you fully explain the indications for and how to use any PRN medication, particularly when to use a GTN spray or salbutamol inhaler
  - Discuss any important side effects, particularly if you need the patient to report any adverse events, e.g. jaundice while on TB therapy
- Try to ascertain if anything precipitated this admission, e.g. recent acquisition of a long-haired cat in the household of a patient presenting with acute asthma
- Address any lifestyle issues that may be negatively impacting the condition, e.g. smoking, weight, high alcohol use
- Formulate a plan of action with the patient
- Reiterate your discussion with the patient to ensure their understanding
- Offer further information sources, e.g. leaflets, societies or groups
- Organize appropriate follow-up
- Close the interview

Tips
- Read the case scenario carefully and structure your interview in 5 minutes beforehand. Jot down the headings and take them into the room as an aide mémoire:
  - Explanation of condition
  - Discussion of regular and PRN medications
  - Side effects
  - Lifestyle
  - Follow-Up
  - Leaflets
- This is a role-play station so use your imagination
- If you are asked a question by the patient and you do not know the answer, say that you are unable to answer at present, but you will find out next time (as you would in real life!)
- Be aware of possible legal and ethical facets to the case and pre-empt the examiners by tackling them in the case before the discussion
- Remember that body language speaks volumes

Breaking bad news
- If done well this can help the patient come to terms with their illness and minimize psychological distress
- There are no hard-and-fast rules, but a patient-centred approach often helps

Approach to the discussion
- Choose a setting that is private and free from disturbance (give your bleep to someone else). Have enough time to do it properly
- Invite other healthcare workers, e.g. a nurse, for support and to ensure continuity of information given by all the team
- Introduce yourself and the purpose of the discussion
- Offer the opportunity for relatives to attend if the patient wishes. This is useful for patient support and can help the dissemination of information
- Check the patient's existing awareness and gauge how much they want to be told
- Give the bad news clearly and simply:
  - Avoid medical jargon
  - Avoid information overload
  - Avoid 'loose terminology' that may be misinterpreted
- Pause and acknowledge distress. Wait for the patient to guide the conversation and explore their concerns as they arise
- If you are unsure as to exact treatment options available, inform the patient that their case is going to be discussed at an MDT (be it cancer or other disease group) and a decision made at that meeting as to best care. Arrange to meet them immediately after this meeting
- Recap what has been discussed and check understanding
- Bring the discussion to a close, but offer an opportunity to speak again and elicit the help of other groups, e.g. specialist cancer nurses or societies, to help the patient at this difficult time
- Enquire how the patient is planning on getting home
  - If they are distressed, advise them that they should not drive
  - Offer to ring a relative to collect them or to arrange a taxi home

Other problems
- **Denial:** If a patient is in denial, reiterate the key message that needs to be addressed
  - Confront the inconsistencies in their perceptions and if this does not work, acknowledge their denial in a sensitive way
  - It may be better to leave this to a later date, perhaps when the patient is ready to confront the painful reality
- **Anger:** This is a natural and usually transient part of the grieving process
  - 'Shooting the messenger' can occur occasionally, particularly if the news is delivered poorly
  - Acknowledge the patient's anger and empathize with their plight
  - If this does not diffuse the situation, terminate the session and reconvene later
- **'How long have I got?':** Explore why the patient wants to know. Answer in broad terms: hours–days, days–weeks, etc.

Points for the exam
- Use real days of the week for the MDT and a date for the follow-up appointment: 'We have our meeting at 8 am on Wednesday morning. I will contact you after this and then see you in the clinic on Thursday 10 June at 3 pm.'

Dealing with a difficult patient

- These are challenging cases but sadly all too common in clinical practice and so will appear in the exam
- A cool head is needed – don't get flustered
- Stay focused

Approach to the discussion

AN ANGRY PATIENT

- Listen without interruption and let them voice their anger
- Keep calm and do not raise your voice
- Acknowledge they are angry and try to explore why
- Empathize by stating that you understand why they are upset, but try to avoid saying that you 'know how they feel'
- Apologize if there has been an error
- Volunteer that if they wish to take matters further that they could contact the Patient Advice and Liaison Service or give them information about the trust's complaints procedure. Most trusts have a leaflet with this information on it

A NON-COMPLIANT PATIENT

- Explore why they have not taken their medication:
  - Were the side effects bothering them?
  - Was the drug not working?
- Educate the patient – perhaps they were not aware how important it was to take the tablets
- Offer solutions:
  - Direct supervision of treatment, e.g. anti-tuberculosis treatment
  - Offer to change the therapy if possible

A SELF-DISCHARGING PATIENT

- Explain why you do not want them to leave
- If they have capacity, they may leave, but they do so at their own risk and against medical advice. To attempt to stop them is assault
- If they lack capacity to make this decision they can be detained by reasonable force, acting in their best interests under common law. To let them go is negligent
  - You may also wish to seek advice with regard to holding them under Section 5.2 of the Mental Health Act while their capacity to make decisions is more formally assessed
  - If in attempting to detain such a person there is risk of serious injury to the patient or those restraining the patient, then you may have no alternative but to let them go
  - If you are presented with this scenario, in the discussion make it clear to the examiners that you would phone the GP and also attempt to contact relatives of the patient to inform them of the events and that the patient might be at risk
- Patients with smear-positive TB (AFBs present in sputum and therefore posing a risk of infection to the public) can be detained, but not treated, under the Public Health Act

A PATIENT THAT CONTINUES TO DRIVE DESPITE CONTRAINDICATION

- Although it is the duty of the patient (not the doctor) to declare a disability that precludes them from holding a UK driving licence, it is one of the acknowledged circumstances (stated by the GMC) under which a breach of confidentiality may be justified
- Try to persuade the patient to inform the DVLA
  - Mention lack of insurance cover if they drive and safety issues to themselves and other road users
  - They can also face a £1000 fine if they do not inform the DVLA of a listed medical condition

- Ask them to provide written evidence that they have informed the DVLA if you suspect they have not
- Inform the patient that you will write to the DVLA if they fail to do so
- Write to the DVLA if no evidence is forthcoming and to the patient to inform them you have done so
- Driving regulations change regularly. It is difficult to give individualized information to patients, especially when an HGV licence is at risk. The information in the table is a guide to current regulations

Driving restrictions

Disease	Private vehicle licence	HGV/PSV licence
First unprovoked seizure with a low rate of recurrence	**6 months** if fit free/medical review **6 months** during treatment changes	**10 years** if risk of recurrence is <2% per annum
Epilepsy (2 or more seizures)	**1 year** if fit free/medical review	**10 years** if fit free off medication
Acute coronary syndrome	**1 month** if untreated **1 week** if treated with stent and it was successful	**6 weeks** if symptom free and cleared by a medical professional
Syncope	**4 weeks** (single with cause, treated) **6 months** (single, unexplained) **12 months** (multiple)	**3 months** (single with cause, treated) **12 months** (single, unexplained) **5 years** (multiple)
Stroke/TIA	**1 month** if no persistent deficit	**1 year** if no persistent deficit
IDDM	**Notify DVLA** may drive if no visual impairment and aware of hypoglycaemia	Will require medical assessment by DVLA

- Any illness where the doctor feels that the patient's ability to drive is significantly impaired should be referred to the DVLA for further action and the patient should be told not to drive in the meantime
- **Other issues to address:**
  - Explore the impact on the patient's job and lifestyle
  - How is the patient going to get home from your clinic? For full guidelines see http://www.dvla.gov.uk/medical/ataglance.aspx

WORKED EXAMPLES

Duty of candour/medical mistake

A 65-year-old man was admitted with new-onset atrial fibrillation that was leading to haemodynamic compromise. On admission he was on warfarin for a metallic mitral valve. His usual dose was 2 mg once a day, but you accidentally prescribed 5 mg once a day for two days. His INR went up to 7. There was no bleeding as a consequence of the high INR. You have been asked to speak with him.

Approach to the discussion
- Duty of candour – responsibility to be honest with patients, colleagues and your organisation when something goes wrong
- Mention that you have only just found out about this – the patient must be informed as soon as possible after the event has occurred
- Bear in mind the welfare of the patient– do they have adequate support around them to receive this information? Are you delivering this information in an appropriate setting?
- Say you are sorry – this does not amount to an admission of negligence or liability (Compensation Act 2006); good medical practice advises that you should say sorry even if you are not the one who has made the mistake
- Ask the patient whether or not they wish to hear the details of the mistake
- Explain what has happened in language that the patient can understand
- Ensure that you explain any immediate and longer-term consequences of the mistake and what has been done to mitigate any issues
- Ask whether the patient has any concerns raised by this news and address those appropriately
- Offer to follow up this apology with a written apology
- State that you have documented the apology in the medical record
- Explain that you have completed a form to trigger an investigation into the mistake by your hospital so that lessons can be learnt from this error to try to prevent it happening again
- Offer information about how to report this to the Patient Advice and Liaison Service

Legal issues
- GMC good medical practice instructs all healthcare professionals that they must have duty of candour after a mistake or near miss has occurred
- If the mistake has resulted in the death of a patient, or led to the patient being in a coma, you are encouraged to speak to the relatives of the patient. Good medical practice encourages the doctor to consider any known views of the patient when speaking with relatives
- All events must be reported through the incident reporting system of the hospital where the event has taken place, but you may also consider reporting to the national Learn from Patient Safety Events service or reporting an adverse outcome following administration of an appropriately prescribed medication through the Yellow Card scheme

Advanced care planning

You are in a neurology clinic reviewing a 58-year-old man with motor neurone disease. He has recently been started on nocturnal non-invasive ventilation. He wishes to speak to you about drawing up an advanced care plan. He has come to the clinic alone. What advice do you offer him?

Approach to the discussion
- Explore whether there are any triggers that have led to him wanting to draw up an advanced care plan
- Ask him about his current symptoms and concerns

- Briefly consider reviewing his mood, paying particular attention to any depressive symptoms or any cues suggesting he may self-harm
- Address those before moving on to discuss the advanced care plan
- Consider his welfare at all times:
  - Does he want someone else to be with him while he is discussing this?
  - Does he wish for his views to be documented now or rather discuss what might go into such a document and have a think about his decisions for them to be documented at a later date?
- Give him information about how to go about drawing up an advanced care plan; explain the legalities of this and what sort of information it should contain
- Check that the patient has capacity to express his wishes and is not being influenced by any external pressures
- If he wishes to compile the advanced care plan now, tell him that you will document it in his medical records
- Ask consent to share it with other healthcare professionals, e.g. GP, ambulance staff
- Encourage him to discuss his plans with his next of kin/family
- At the end of the discussion recap what you have discussed and in particular address what you are going to do to help with any new symptoms
- State that you will re-review the plan with him at the next clinic appointment to check that he hasn't changed his mind about any of the issues documented
- At the end again think about his welfare:
  - 'We have discussed some difficult topics this morning. Are you OK to get home?'
  - 'Would you like to sit in the waiting room to gather your thoughts before leaving the hospital?'

Legal issues
- An advanced care plan is drawn up to help patients document their medical wishes as they approach the end of their life
  - It can be particularly useful when it is anticipated that a patient may lose the ability to communicate their wishes or lose the capacity to make decisions
- It does not need to be witnessed by a legal professional, but it is advisable that it is discussed with healthcare professionals and family members at the time that it is formulated
- The types of decisions that might be included in the document can range from specific medical treatments, e.g. not to be ventilated or resuscitated, to more general wishes such as the patient would wish to be given access to palliative care or a wish to die in a hospice or at home if possible
- If the patient states that they would want a specific treatment in the future, you would need to inform them that it might not be possible to offer that treatment in the future, but that their wishes will certainly be taken into account
- The patient should be aware that they are at liberty to update this document at any time and that if any of the scenarios documented arise, then the doctor looking after the patient will check with them that they still hold those same views and haven't changed their mind
- If you live in the UK, prior to the exam check if the region you live in has signed up to the Resus Council's ReSPECT (Recommended Summary Plan for Emergency Care and treatment) programme. This is a way of documenting and sharing any advanced decisions patients have made about their wishes for their management in an emergency, e.g. cardiac arrest at home

Advanced decisions to refuse treatment
- Advanced decisions to refuse treatment (ADRT), previously known as advanced directives, can be written by a person who has capacity and who wishes to express decisions to refuse treatment in the future, should they lose the ability to express their wishes or lose the capacity to make decisions

- The ADRT can be verbally expressed to a third party, but it is best if it is a written document signed by a witness. This witness does not need to be a solicitor or other professional and can be a family member
- It is recommended that:
  - The document contains the name and address of the individual expressing their wishes
  - The name and address of their GP
  - The document is dated
  - The wishes of the individual are clearly documented, including the circumstances in which the decision would apply
  - If the decision is to refuse a life-saving or life-sustaining treatment, such as antibiotics for pneumonia, the phrase 'even if life is at risk' is documented
  - A copy is forwarded to the individual's GP
- A doctor can be at risk of battery if he/she does not comply with the wishes expressed in a ADRT document. The doctor needs to be satisfied that the individual had capacity at the time of the writing of the document, that they were free of coercion at that time and that they fully understood the consequences of their wishes

Needlestick injury

A 28-year-old phlebotomist working in your hospital sustained a needlestick injury following taking blood from a patient. The patient has now left the hospital. The patient has not previously been tested for any blood-borne viruses. You have been asked to see the phlebotomist in the Accident and Emergency Department as part of the medical take. It is 2 pm. Counsel the phlebotomist about any complications that might arise. What further management would you advise?

Approach to the discussion

- Ascertain the details of the incident; check that the needle had actually been used to take blood from the patient prior to the needlestick injury
- Ensure that the phlebotomist has completed the following steps:
  - Disposed of the needle
  - Encouraged the wound to bleed
  - Washed the wound with water for a minimum of 60 seconds
  - Placed a plaster over the site of the needlestick injury
- Explain that the risk of being infected with a blood-borne virus from a needlestick injury is very low:
  - 1 in 3 for hepatitis B if unvaccinated
  - 1 in 30 for hepatitis C
  - 1 in 300 for HIV
- Ask if the phlebotomist has the patient's details as well as the name of the doctor who referred the patient for a blood test
- Ask if the phlebotomist has had hepatitis B vaccinations previously
- Consent the phlebotomist for a blood sample for pre-existing hepatitis and HIV; explain that the results will be treated confidentially and only shared with their direct-care clinical team and that they have the right to refuse to be tested
- If the phlebotomist has not previously been given hepatitis B vaccination, then offer rapid immunization
- Explain that post-exposure prophylaxis (PEP) for HIV may be required. The first dose of PEP should be administered within 72 h but is most effective if taken within 24 h of exposure
- Explain that the phlebotomist should contact occupational health immediately as the incident has taken place within office hours. They will consent the patient for a blood sample to test for viruses
- If the patient cannot be found or does not wish to consent to be tested, then PEP may be considered
- Encourage the phlebotomist to complete an incident form

Epilepsy

An 18-year-old woman who is trying to become a professional model has had her second general-ized seizure in three months, which was witnessed by her GP. She has had a normal CT head and metabolic causes have been excluded. She has returned to your outpatient clinic for the results. Please discuss the diagnosis with her.

Approach to the discussion

- The diagnosis is epilepsy. Explain what this means to the patient in lay terms: 'disorganized electrical activity in the brain' (see Information Delivery)
- Explore **social aspects:**
  - She has been drinking a lot of alcohol recently and staying out late at all-night parties
  - She drives to modelling agencies and relies heavily on her car
  - She hates taking tablets
- Discuss **treatment** options to limit her seizure activity:
  - Avoid excess alcohol and sleep deprivation
  - Avoid precipitants, e.g. flashing disco lights
  - Drugs: there are some newer anti-epileptic medications, e.g. lamotrigine, that have fewer side effects. This is important to her as she is a model
- Stress **compliance** (if poor compliance see Dealing with a Difficult Patient):
  - It is imperative that if she is on the oral contraceptive combined pill, she is told the risks of **pill failure**. This is important, as anti-epileptics are teratogenic
  - Advise alternative forms of contraception, e.g. barrier, or if this is unacceptable switch to a higher-dose oestrogen pill or progesterone pill
  - If she wants to become **pregnant,** it is a balance of risk between a seizure when pregnant, which carries a significant risk of miscarriage, and the potential teratogenic side effects of the drugs
  - Most physicians encourage female patients wishing to start a family to continue on their epileptic treatment. Remember folate supplements
- **Safety** issues:
  - Avoid swimming or bathing alone and heights
  - Driving restrictions (if she continues to drive see Dealing with a Difficult Patient and Breaking Confidentiality)
- **Recap** the important points and formulate an agreed plan
- **Check understanding** and answer her questions
- **Other information:** offer leaflets, British Epilepsy Society (www.epilepsy.org.uk) contact numbers and an appointment with an epilepsy specialist nurse
- Conclude the interview after ascertaining how she is going to get home

Huntington's chorea

A 26-year-old son of your patient has requested to see you to discuss his mother's diagnosis. She has developed a dementing illness and chorea in her late 40s. Her father committed suicide at the age of 60. A diagnosis of Huntington's chorea has been made on genetic testing. She currently lives in her own home but is not coping. She has also asked her son to help her die. Discuss the relevant issues with her son. He and his partner are planning to have children.

Approach to the discussion

- Ascertain that his mother has consented to this discussion, to avoid the **confidentiality** pitfall and a rather short interview
  - Remember if the mother is your patient and the son is not, you only have a duty of care to the mother
  - If she does not want you to discuss the diagnosis with her son, then to do so would breach confidentiality

- Explain Huntington's chorea and its inheritance to the son (see Information Delivery and Breaking Bad News). Emphasize that there is **no cure** and management is supportive
- Explore how the diagnosis **relates to him** and his family:
  - Anticipation, i.e. if he is affected the onset may be at an earlier age
  - Genetic screening and family planning
  - Prenatal screening. This would potentially result in an abortion – briefly explore this with the patient
- Life insurance and employment implications.
- Explain how the diagnosis **relates to his mother:**
  - Social aspects: community care or nursing home placement plans
  - Legal aspects: advanced decisions to refuse treatment (previously known as advanced directives), lasting power of attorney may be discussed (see Competence and Consent**)**
  - Assisted suicide is illegal (see End-of-Life Decisions)
- **Recap** and formulate an agreed plan
- **Check understanding** and answer questions
- **Other information:**
  - Offer leaflets, Huntington's society contact numbers and an appointment with a geneticist
  - An appointment with a social worker would be useful to organize residential care for his mother
- **Arrange follow-up,** ideally with all the family as it affects all of them
- Conclude the interview

Tips for the exam
- This is a complex question and a candidate could lose marks by not covering all the points raised in the scenario
- Make notes in the 5 minutes before you go into the station with headings to include:
  - Consent
  - Explanation of Huntington's disease
  - Care of the mother
  - Impact of diagnosis on son, his future children and any other family members
  - How to manage the request to help her die
- Watch the clock, as one could easily spend the allotted time just covering the genetic aspects of this scenario

Paracetamol overdose
A patient arrives in the emergency medical unit having taken 50 paracetamol tablets 4 hours ago. She says she wants to die and does not want to be treated, although she would like painkillers for her abdominal pain. Negotiate a treatment plan with this patient.

Approach to the discussion
- Be clear on the amount of paracetamol taken and the time of ingestion as this will influence the management, i.e. calculating the treatment level of paracetamol
- Alcoholism or anti-epileptic medication lowers the treatment line
- Assess the suicidal intent, e.g. letter
- Discuss previous psychiatric history
- Negotiate an agreed **treatment plan** if possible
- Organize a referral to the deliberate self-harm team
- **Recap** and **check understanding**
- Conclude the interview

Legal issues: treatment debate
- **Competency:**
  - Does she understand that this overdose is life-threatening and what the treatment involves?
  - Is the paracetamol overdose affecting her judgement?
  - Is a psychiatric illness affecting her judgement, e.g. is she delusional?
- If she is deemed to lack capacity, then you must act in her best interests and treat her against her will under **common law**
- If she has capacity, she has a right to refuse treatment
- If you do not treat and the patient dies, you may have to defend this decision in court
  - If you treat her in the face of her wishes, you could be charged with battery
  - Most courts will not find physicians that act in the patient's best interests guilty
- **Implied consent:** This may be invoked to defend treatment of a patient who arrives in hospital having taken an overdose, but they may have been taken there against their will, or they may have attended hospital to palliate their symptoms
- **Advanced decision to refuse treatment:** Notes stating they do not wish to be treated may be ignored, because the attending physician often cannot be sure of the circumstances in which they were written, e.g. under duress, or that the patient has not changed her mind
- **The Mental Health Act** cannot be invoked to treat overdose patients, even if they have depression
- Attempted suicide is no longer illegal in the UK
  - Assisting someone to commit suicide *is* illegal
- If in doubt, it is prudent to treat overdose patients under common law, acting in their best interests
  - It may be advisable to seek legal advice

Brain-stem death and organ donation
You are working in intensive care and you have recently admitted a 30-year-old man who was hit by a car. He has sustained a severe head injury and his second assessment of brain-stem function shows he is brain-stem dead. You have found an organ donor card in his wallet. Please discuss the diagnosis with his mother and father and broach the subject of organ donation with them.

Approach to the discussion
BRAIN-STEM DEATH
- Explain that he has had a severe brain injury and that he is brain dead (see Breaking Bad News)
- Inform them about brain-stem death:
  - 'He has died and only the ventilator is keeping his other organs working'
- Pause for reflection and questions

ORGAN DONATION
- Broach the subject in a sensitive way
- Explain that while he is brain dead his other organs are working well and are suitable for donation
- If he is not registered as opting out of donation, did he express any wishes prior to this event?
- Points that can be addressed may include:
  - The need for **an operation** to 'harvest' the organs
  - **HIV testing** prior to donation
  - Not all the organs taken may be used
  - Time delays involved prior to the certification of death and the release of the body

- Avoid information overload and be guided by the relative's questions and the time available
- Offer to put them in touch with the **transplant coordinator** for the region, who will be able to counsel them further
- Remind them that a decision has to be made swiftly, but avoid harassing the relatives unduly (offer to come back when they have had a chance to think about it)
- Being too involved in the transplantation program may be ethically wrong for an ITU physician, due to potentially conflicting interests
- **Recap** and formulate a plan
- **Check understanding** at each stage and answer their questions
- **Offer other information:** leaflet on transplantation
- Conclude the interview

Tip for the exam
- Completing this scenario well hinges on whether you are able to explain to the family about brain-stem death
- This is best approached as if you are breaking news that the patient has died. It avoids ambiguity as to whether or not there is any chance of recovery

BRAIN-STEM DEATH AND ORGAN DONATION
- Discussion with a coroner must occur prior to organ donation if it is a coroner's case
- Permission may be withheld if a death is due to a criminal action
- **Donation after brain death** (DBD) involves donation of organs after the patient meets criteria for death by neurological criteria
- **Donation after cardiac death** (DCD) involves donation of organs after irreversible cessation of circulatory and respiratory function

HUMAN TISSUE ACT 1961 AND HUMAN ORGAN TRANSPLANT ACT 1989
- Statute law defines codes of practice on organ retrieval, consent and diagnostic tests of brain death
- To establish brain-stem death two consultants assess independently that:
  - The cause of death is known and all potentially treatable causes for the patient's state have been excluded, e.g. hypothermia, biochemical derangement and drugs, i.e. the unconscious state is **irreversible** and **permanent**
  - The brain stem reflexes, e.g. pupil, corneal, motor cranial nerve responses, vestibulo-ocular, gag and cough reflexes, are absent and there is no spontaneous respiratory drive at a $PaCO_2$ >50 mm Hg

ORGAN DONATION LAW IN THE UK
- Organ donation law has changed in all areas of the UK in the last five years
- Broadly speaking it is now an opt-out system across the UK for all adults
- There are subtle differences across the devolved nations with regard to the terms used and importantly the age of the patient
- **England:**
  - Opt-out system – assumed consent unless you opt out on the UK Organ donation website
  - Aged >18 years old
  - Excluded groups:
    - Those lacking mental capacity
    - Those who have been living in England for <12 months
    - Visitors to England
    - Those not living in England voluntarily
- **Wales:**
  - 'Deemed consent' – assumed consent unless you opt out on the UK Organ donation website

- o Can nominate two people to make decisions on your behalf
- o Aged >18 years old
- o Excluded groups:
  - o Those lacking mental capacity
  - o Those who have been living in Wales for <12 months
  - o Visitors to Wales
- **Scotland:**
  - o 'Deemed authorization' – assumed consent unless you opt out on the UK Organ donation website
  - o Aged >16 years old
  - o Excluded groups:
    - o Those lacking mental capacity
    - o Those who have been living in Scotland for <12 months
    - o Visitors to Scotland
- **Northern Ireland:**
  - o Opt-out system – assumed consent unless you opt out on the UK Organ donation website
  - o Aged >18 years old
  - o Excluded groups:
    - o Those lacking mental capacity
    - o Those who have been living in Northern Ireland for <12 months
    - o Visitors to Northern Ireland

Non-compliant diabetic

A 26-year-old female insulin-dependent diabetic has been admitted with yet another ketoacidotic episode. She has family problems. You notice she is very thin and has lanugo hair on her face. Please counsel her regarding her poor diabetic control and weight loss.

Approach to the discussion
- **Diabetic education:**
  - o Review insulin regimen, injection sites and **compliance** (may be non-compliant due to weight gain or family problems)
  - o Educate about the importance of tight glycaemic control and the dangers of diabetic ketoacidosis
  - o Ask about other cardiovascular risk factors, e.g. smoking
- **Dieting and anorexia nervosa:**
  - o Emphasize the importance of a balanced diet and diabetic control
  - o Explore her dietary intake
  - o Ask her about her weight, body image and self-esteem
  - o Assess for **depression** (associated with anorexia)
- **Family problems:**
  - o Explore these and counsel as required
  - o Patients suffering from anorexia often have problems at home
  - o **Family therapy** can be useful in treating anorexia nervosa
- **Recap** and formulate a plan
- **Check understanding** and answer questions
- **Offer other information:** leaflets and Anorexia Nervosa Society details
- Conclude the interview

Legal issues
- **Capacity:** due to the effects of malnutrition on cognition, an anorexic patient may not be competent to refuse treatment
- Anorexia nervosa can be treated under the **Mental Health Act 1983** as an outpatient or in severe cases on a specialist unit
- Food is deemed a treatment for a mental illness and can be given against the patient's will under the Mental Health Act

Vaccination compliance

A 32-year-old woman is admitted under the medical take with increased shortness of breath. She is 8 weeks pregnant. She has a history of asthma and is currently treated with combination inhaled corticosteroid and long-acting β-agonist. She has a reduced peak flow rate and auscultation of her chest reveals inspiratory wheeze. Her Wells score is 0 and her D-dimer is negative despite the pregnancy. She has never had an influenza vaccination and is not up to date with her Covid-19 vaccinations.

Approach to the discussion

- Start by explaining that she has had an exacerbation of her asthma and what treatment you are going to offer her
- Give her an opportunity early on to express any concerns that she might have
- Reassure her that this will not affect the development of the baby
- Try to ascertain briefly if there were any potential triggers to this exacerbation – remember this is not a history-taking station
- Check that she is not smoking
- Spend the majority of the time on discussing vaccination, as there is good evidence that both flu and Covid-19 vaccination protect both mother and baby during pregnancy – recommended by the Royal College of Obstetricians and also the Joint Committee on Vaccination and Immunisation
- Influenza vaccination:
  - Decreases the risk of premature or low birthweight babies and still birth
  - Also protects the mother from pneumonitis
  - It is not a live vaccine and is safe to be administered during pregnancy from the first few weeks until delivery
  - Passes on some protection to the baby
  - Can be given at the same time as the whooping cough vaccination, which is usually administered to pregnant women between 16 and 32 weeks
- Covid-19 vaccination:
  - Medical studies have proven it is safe and useful in pregnant women
  - 250,000 pregnant women have now been vaccinated with no concern over safety to the mother or the baby and lower rates of infection in vaccinated pregnant women, similar rates of hospitalization but lower supplemental oxygen requirements and reduced need for vasopressors if needing ITU admission
  - If the pregnant woman has received a full course of immunization with a recent booster, there is significant protection in comparison with those who received the initial two vaccinations in 2020/2021: 88% less likely to need admission to hospital, decreased rates of pre-term birth, lower rates of very low birthweight babies and still birth, and decreased rates of admission to ITU
  - No concerns with regard to breast feeding with either flu or Covid-19 vaccines
  - mRNA vaccines do not cross the placenta (tested in samples taken from human cord blood)
  - Current Covid-19 vaccines include a combination of protection against earlier variants as well as Omicron
  - Side effects with the vaccination are similar in pregnant and non-pregnant women – painful arm, feeling tired, headache, generalized aches and pains
  - Serious side effects with the Covid-19 vaccine include myocarditis, but this has been mainly seen in younger men rather than women

Tips for the exam

- Remember this station is there for you to demonstrate that you can communicate well, exhibit good clinical knowledge and judgement, while also actively listening to the patient's concerns and maintaining their welfare at all times

- Avoid turning it into a consultation station about the asthma
- Impart the appropriate information with regard to vaccinations and ensure that you have informed the patient about the significant benefits to her and her unborn child
- Your role is to ensure that you have informed the patient of the facts for her to then make the best decision for her and her unborn baby. Your role is not to force her to have a vaccination
- In the final two minutes, ensure that you have agreed a plan for her asthma follow-up and also a plan with regard to the vaccinations, e.g. she is going to discuss this further with her obstetrician, discuss with friends and family or she is happy to book one through the NHS vaccines booking system

Shared decision making

A 48-year-old man developed an idiopathic pulmonary embolism nine months ago. He has presented to A&E today with an ankle injury that he sustained while at work as a builder. During a follow-up conversation, he stated that he had stopped his apixaban a few weeks ago without seeking medical advice first. The A&E team have asked you as the medical team on call to discuss this with him.

Approach to the discussion

- Briefly go over the circumstances of the PE – take care not to turn this into a history-taking station
- Check that he is back to full health following the event – if he is still breathless, he may require investigation for chronic thromboembolic disease, which will alter the recommendations regarding long-term anticoagulation
- Explore the reasons behind why he chose to stop taking the medication:
  - Was he worried about bleeding risk?
  - Does he play contact sports?
- Explain that your role is to ensure that the patient has the necessary information to make a decision that is right for him and that your job is not to tell him what he must do
- Explain that there is concern that if there are no identifiable provoking factors for a PE then there is a significant annual risk of recurrence of the PE
- Decisions about prolonged anticoagulation focus on the risk of recurrence versus the risk of bleeding plus the individual's lifestyle and personal beliefs
- The only provoking factors deemed low risk are:
  - Surgery with GA for >30 min
  - Trauma with fracture to bones
  - Strict bed rest in hospital for >3 days (ESC PE Guidelines 2019)
- If no provoking factors annual risk of further PE is ~4.5%
- Some studies have also suggested that male sex and an idiopathic VTE event in patients under 50 years old also increase the risk of recurrence
- Can also measure D-dimer in this context to add into the algorithm of risk
  - If it continues to be elevated three months after the acute event then the risk is increased
- The risk of bleeding can be assessed using the HAS-BLED score, which includes parameters such as presence of systemic hypertension, renal impairment, age >65, previous history of a CVA, use of other medication such as aspirin and also drinking >8 units of alcohol per week
  - If alcohol use is the only risk factor, then the annual bleed is about 1 patient per 100 per year will have a bleed
- Andexanet alfa is a recombinant form of Factor Xa that acts an antidote to both apixaban and rivaroxaban and is in the BNF

- ○ It has a conditional marketing authorization at present but can be considered for use in life-threatening or uncontrolled bleeding
- ○ A decision from NICE re its use is expected in 2025–2026
- Finally, you could offer for him to be seen by a haematologist

Tips for the exam
- Explore the patient's concerns and actively address any questions he has
- Do not feel under pressure to change the patient's mind
- Your role is to provide the information, make sure that he is not harbouring any misinformation and answer any questions that he has with your knowledge of the evidence as it stands

Sample questions for self-directed learning

Information delivery

- A 60-year-old man is about to leave hospital, 7 days after an uncomplicated MI. He has some concerns regarding his return to normal life. He has been commenced on standard secondary prophylaxis for ischaemic heart disease. What advice would you give him regarding his condition?
- A 23-year-old newly diagnosed asthmatic has been recently discharged from hospital and arrives in your outpatient clinic for a review of his illness. He works as a veterinary nurse and smokes 15 cigarettes per day. Educate him about his illness, arrange further tests and instigate a treatment plan.
- A 32-year-old woman has been recently diagnosed with multiple sclerosis following a second episode of optic neuritis. Discuss her diagnosis, prognosis and likely treatment options.
- A 29-year-old man with a 14-year history of ulcerative colitis treated with steroids and ciclosporin has come to your follow-up clinic. He is concerned with some of the side effects he has been having on his medication. Address this and counsel him in the further management of his condition.
- A 50-year-old heavy smoker presents with his fifth exacerbation of COPD this year. He tells you he does not take his inhalers because he thinks they make him worse. His blood gas on air reads a PaO_2 of 6.8 kPa. Discuss treatment options with him.

Communicating medico-legal and ethical principles

A patient with metastatic breast carcinoma attends your clinic. She has read on the internet that there is a new treatment that might be helpful. Unfortunately, your Trust has decided not to fund this treatment at present. Counsel her on these matters.

- A patient's relatives arrive to be told that their father was unfortunately dead on arrival at hospital. It is likely he suffered a large myocardial infarction. Break this bad news to them and guide them with regard to the need for a coroner's postmortem. For religious reasons they would like the body released today.
- A 90-year-old woman who has recently had a debilitating stroke has a GCS of 7/15. A decision has been made to put in place a 'do not attempt resuscitation' order. Her daughter has arrived on the ward and would like to speak to a doctor. Discuss the management of this patient with the daughter.
- A 53-year-old woman with end-stage renal failure has been admitted. She gives you a list of situations in which she does not wish to be treated, including commencing dialysis. Discuss the advanced directive for refusal of treatment with her and assess whether or not you think it is appropriate to comply with the document.
- A 49-year-old man is admitted to Accident and Emergency with a complete left-sided pneumothorax. He has a history of COPD. Consent him for insertion of a chest drain.

Consultations

Clinical mark sheet

Clinical skill	Satisfactory	Unsatisfactory
Physical examination	Correct, thorough, fluent, systematic, professional	Incorrect technique, omits, unsystematic, hesitant
Identifying physical signs	Identifies correct signs Does not find signs that are not present	Misses important signs Finds signs that are not present
Clinical communication skills	Elicits appropriate and relevant history, assesses impact on patient and patient's preferences Explains clinical information that is accurate, clear, structured, comprehensive, fluent, professional	Omits important areas of history, inaccurate, fails to assess impact of symptoms, insufficient, unclear, ambiguous, unstructured, uses jargon, unpractised, does not involve patient/relative in management plan
Differential diagnosis	Constructs sensible differential diagnosis	Poor differential, fails to consider the correct diagnosis
Clinical judgement	Sensible, relevant and appropriate management plan, applies clinical knowledge appropriately, addresses time scales	Inappropriate management Does not apply clinical knowledge to the case
Managing patients' concerns	Seeks, detects and addresses patient's concerns, actively listens, confirms understanding, empathetic	Overlooks concerns, does not address patient's questions, poor listening, not empathetic Does not check understanding
Maintaining patient welfare	Respectful, sensitive Ensures comfort, safety and dignity	Causes physical or emotional discomfort Jeopardizes patient safety

Cases for PACES, Fourth Edition. Stephen Hoole, Andrew Fry and Rachel Davies.
© 2025 John Wiley & Sons Ltd. Published 2025 by John Wiley & Sons Ltd.

Consultation – general advice

- This station is designed to bring everything together and assesses all seven skills in a way that most accurately reflects real clinical practice
- It assesses the approach of the candidate to clinical scenarios that are frequently encountered on a medical take or in a general medical clinic
- It lends itself to cases that are multisystemic and have a multidisciplinary focus. Subspecialty cases that do not feature in other stations (e.g. skin, locomotor, haematological and endocrine cases) can appear here too
- This station is often the hardest to master within the short 15-minute time allowed
  - Examiners are looking to pass candidates who are not fazed by complexity and who can ask pertinent questions and elicit diagnostic clinical signs that focus on the key important features of a case
  - Responding to the clinical features of the case as they emerge and thinking on your feet is encouraged
  - Passing this station will demonstrate efficient and effective practice that is required to cope with a busy acute medical take or overrunning outpatient clinic. Spending time in these departments will help you prepare
- You will have some preparation time before this station when you will be given the candidate information for the scenario to read
  - Use this preparatory time wisely by listing the diagnosis/differential diagnoses and the key features of the history and examination that you plan to elicit during the cases
- You then have 15 minutes to assess the patient (with a bell 1 minute before the end) and then 5 minutes for discussion with the examiners to justify your differential diagnosis and formulate a management plan
  - It is imperative that history and examination are performed as both carry marks
  - There is not much time, but do not forget the basics: introduce yourself, be empathetic and maintain patient welfare. These are also assessed
  - Considering the patient's 'lived experience' of the disease is important and remember that management should always include advice, sources of information and support
- Be systematic and efficient, utilising open and closed questioning during history taking as the time allows
- Be flexible and respond empathetically to your patient's concerns, but be in control, the clock is ticking!
- Use non-verbal cues, for example by standing or holding the patient's hand as a prompt to seek their permission to examine them. This will indicate to even the most talkative patient that history taking is complete and sensitively signposts to them that you politely want to move on with the examination
- Cases encountered in this section fall into two broad categories, both of which we include in this chapter:
  - Symptomatic presentations with a broad differential diagnosis (e.g. chest pain or dyspnoea – we have highlighted the key diagnostic symptoms/signs and results in bold)
  - Specific conditions that are often multisystem disorders (e.g. the patient with obvious systemic sclerosis)
- For all the cases we list pertinent points to elicit from the history, important examination findings and discussion topics that may be encountered
- This approach is not exhaustive and is intended as a guide – you may decide that other aspects of a similar case deserve more attention on the day, particularly if the patient raises them with you; let the patient be your guide on what to focus on

Chest pain
This 54-year-old male smoker has chest pain. Please can you assess him.

- **Diagnosis:** myocardial ischaemia
- **Differential diagnosis:** pleuritic (PE or pneumonia), pericarditic, musculoskeletal, oesophageal reflux/spasm

History
ESTABLISH SYMPTOM IS ANGINA
- Character: **dull ache**, band-like and tightness
- Position/**radiation:** substernal into **arm/jaw**
- Exacerbating and relieving factors:
  - ↑ Heavy meals, cold, **exertion** and emotional stress
  - ↓ Rest and/or sublingual GTN (although may relieve oesophageal spasm as well)
- Associated symptoms: nausea, sweating and breathlessness
- Differential diagnosis: pleuritic chest pain or cough (lung), viral illnesses/prodrome (pericarditis), history of peptic ulcers (GI), recent heavy lifting (musculoskeletal)

RISK FACTORS FOR CAD
- Smoking, diabetes, family history, cholesterol, ↑BP, age and ethnic origin (South Asian)

IMPACT OF SYMPTOMS ON PROFESSION
- DVLA restrictions

TREATMENT CONSIDERATIONS
- Any contraindications to antiplatelet agents/anticoagulants/thrombolysis, e.g. peptic ulcer
- PVD: femoral and radial pulse for angiography
- Varicose veins: surgical conduits for grafting

Examination
HANDS AND PULSE
- Tar-stained fingers (smoking), pulse rate and rhythm

EYES
- Xanthelasma (cholesterol)

AUSCULTATION
- Heart: murmurs – AS or MR
- Chest bibasal crackles: CCF

PERIPHERIES
- Swollen ankles: CCF

Discussion
INITIAL INVESTIGATIONS
- Acute: 12-lead ECG and CXR, troponin, FBC, creatinine (eGFR), fasting lipid profile and glucose

EMERGENCY TREATMENT (ACS)
- Antithrombotic/antiplatelet; GpIIb/IIIa inhibitor if high risk (TIMI risk score ≥4)
- Antianginal: GTN and β-blocker
- Risk modifiers: statin and ACE inhibitors

- **Invasive coronary angiography** (if troponin positive):
  - Angioplasty and stent
  - Surgery: CABG
  - May require mechanical support with IABP as a bridge to surgical revascularization
- Further investigations (if troponin negative):
  - CTCA or invasive coronary angiography (depending on pre-test probability)
  - Functional tests to confirm ischaemia: exercise stress test, MIBI scan and stress echo or MRI

GRACE AND TIMI RISK SCORES

- Estimate mortality for patients with ACS and are used to triage ACS patients for urgent invasive treatment

ELECTIVE MANAGEMENT (STABLE)

- Lifestyle and risk factor modification. NICE recommends statins in those with 10-year risk of CV event >10%
- Aspirin and antianginal: β-blocker, nitrate, nicorandil, ranolazine, ivabradine, CCB
- **NICE recommends CTCA** in preference to functional imaging initially
- Revascularization (stent or surgery) considered for patients with symptoms of angina that fails to settle on two anti-anginal medications; revascularization has no prognostic benefit in those without significant left main stem disease

REFRACTORY ANGINA

- Chest pain that is not relieved with anti-anginal medication at appropriate dose, stents or bypass surgery
- **Emerging treatments:** coronary sinus reducer, spinal cord stimulator and stellate ganglion block

ANGINA (ISCHAEMIA) NON-OBSTRUCTIVE CORONARY ARTERY (A(I)NOCA)

- **Causes:** coronary microcirculatory dysfunction (CMD) – functional or structural endotypes and coronary vasospasm
- **Investigation:**
  - Stress perfusion CMR
  - Coronary reactivity testing with adenosine and Ach
- **Treatment:**
  - CMD – statin, ACE inhibitor, nebivolol
  - Coronary vasospasm – statin, nitrates and CCB

Pericarditis with effusion
This 34-year-old female has had a viral illness and now has chest pain.

- **Likely diagnosis:** acute pericarditis
- **Differential diagnosis:** pleurisy – acute PE, pneumonia; musculoskeletal; MI

History
- **Pleuritic** chest pain – sharp and worse on deep breathing
- **Positional** – relieved sitting forwards, worse lying back
- **Prodromal viral** illness – cough, sore throat, fatigue, low-grade fever
- Duration: acute (few weeks), recurrent (1–2 months), chronic (>3 months)
- Associated symptoms: palpitations, SOB, dizziness, syncope; abdominal distension
- Causes: viral; HIV/TB, uraemia, cancer, autoimmune disease, e.g. rheumatoid arthritis, lupus, previous trauma/cardiac surgery/MI (post-cardiotomy syndrome/Dressler's)
- Differential diagnosis: cough, SOB (pneumonia); long-haul flight, swollen calf (PE); RFs for IHD (MI)

Examination
- **Pericardial rub** – sounds 'squeaky' like walking in fresh snow
- Tamponade is a clinical diagnosis classically described in Beck's triad: hypotension, JVP elevation/distension and muffled heart sounds. Tachycardia (to maintain cardiac output) is also an early sign
- **Pulsus paradoxus:** SBP drops >10 mm Hg on inspiration
- **Kussmaul's sign:** elevated JVP on inspiration
- Signs of an underlying cause, e.g. rheumatoid hands

Discussion
INVESTIGATIONS
- ECG: **global saddle ST elevation**, PR depression, low voltage (pericardial effusion), electrical alternans (heart swinging about in large effusion), tachycardia
- Bloods: troponin may be elevated in myopericarditis; U&E, Cr, ESR, CRP, autoantibodies
- CXR: globular enlarged cardiac silhouette, associated pleural effusion, lung CA
- **Echo:** bright pericardium, effusion, right atrial systolic and **right ventricular diastolic collapse**, regional wall motion abnormality (myopericarditis)
- **Cardiac MRI: meso- or epicardium LGE** indicates myopericarditis rather than MI
- CT: thickened pericardium
- Diagnostic pericardiocentesis (malignant cells, protein, blood)

TREATMENT
- Acute pericarditis is usually self-limiting
- Anti-inflammatory, e.g. **NSAID** or aspirin; **colchicine** (counsel on side effects – nausea, contraindicated in liver/kidney disease and beware drug interactions)
- Recurrent pericarditis may benefit from corticosteroids
- Tamponade is a medical emergency causing RV collapse and hypotension. Emergency treatment with brisk volume expansion (leg raise, IV fluid) and Imaging-guided **pericardiocentesis**
- Complications of pericardiocentesis: puncture of RV, coronary or internal mammary, pneumothorax, liver laceration
- Chronic/constrictive pericarditis may need surgical pericardiectomy

Atrial fibrillation

This 81-year-old male patient has had intermittent palpitations and breathlessness and noticed transient left facial and upper-arm paraesthesia.

History
- Symptoms of atrial fibrillation:
  - Onset and offset, frequency and duration
  - Breathlessness, chest pain, palpitations, presyncope
  - Precipitants: alcohol, caffeine, exercise
- Associated conditions – particularly important for stroke risk:
  - Cardiac problems: valvular heart disease, IHD (explore risk factors), HF
  - Hypertension
  - Hyperthyroidism – tremor, sweating, weight loss
  - Stroke or TIA (likely in this case)
  - Lung disease including PE
- Treatment considerations:
  - Anticoagulation and risk factors for bleeding: alcohol/NSAIDs; renal failure – dose reduction for NOAC; explore risk–benefit of OAC
  - Assess patient preferences to rate vs rhythm control: anti-arrhythmic vs cardioversion vs ablation (pulmonary vein isolation)

Examination
- Cardiovascular examination:
  - Pulse and BP
  - Auscultation: murmurs – MS or MR
  - Signs of CCF
- Assessment of thyroid status:
  - Tremor
  - Goitre
  - Eye disease: lid lag, exophthalmos (Grave's disease)
- Brief neurological examination:
  - Pronator drift
  - Visual fields
  - CN VII weakness
  - CN V and upper-limb sensation
  - Gait and frailty – falls risk

Discussion
INVESTIGATION
- Confirmation: 12-lead ECG or 24 h Holter monitor or event recorder
- Echo: structural disease, LVH, LA size (>4.0 cm – recurrence high), LVEF
- U&E, Cr, LFTs, TSH, Hb, INR

CATEGORY
- Paroxysmal: <7 days, usually self-terminating within 48 h
- Persistent: >7 days, may require chemical or electrical cardioversion
- Permanent: >1 year or when no further attempts to restore sinus

MANAGEMENT
- Address underlying causes – lifestyle: abstinence alcohol; weight loss
- **Rate control:**
  - β-blockers, rate-limiting CCB
  - Digoxin and pacemaker with AVN ablation (elderly) – irreversible

- **Rhythm control:**
  - Chemical or electrical cardioversion (<48 h onset or OAC for at least 3 weeks or TOE to rule out LAA thrombus) – symptomatic patients, HF caused by AF, young, 'pill in the pocket' for paroxysmal AF (normal LV, SBP >100 mm Hg)
  - AF ablation may be considered after confirming the patient is better in sinus rhythm; more successful in paroxysmal AF (>90% cure rate) and atrial flutter
- **Anticoagulation:**
  - Non-valvular AF – first line: NOACs, or continue warfarin if stable INR, time in therapeutic range (TTR) >65%
  - Valvular AF: warfarin
  - Consider patient preference (shared decision making) and cognitive function, lifestyle (diet and alcohol), drug interactions, compliance, monitoring
- **Risk prediction:**
  - Embolic risk equivalent for paroxysmal, persistent and permanent AF and atrial flutter
  - Do not discontinue OAC if sinus rhythm is achieved (except post-op AF)
  - Treat hypertension, advise avoidance of alcohol/NSAIDs to minimise bleeding risk
  - Personalize care: educate re stroke awareness – FAST, support networks
  - Consider LAAO if OAC contraindicated/intolerance or LAA excision in patients undergoing cardiothoracic surgery
  - In an acute life-threatening bleed, consider antidotes e.g., recombinant factor Xa and mAb to dabigatran (NOACs), FFP or vitamin K (warfarin) and protamine (heparins)

Systemic emboli risk: **CHA2DS2VASC**

C	Congestive cardiac failure = 1
H	Hypertension = 1
A_2	Age ≥75 = 2
D	Diabetes = 1
S_2	Stroke/TIA/embolus = 2
V	Vascular disease = 1
A	Age 65–74 = 1
Sc	Sex category (female) = 1

0 = Low stroke risk = no anticoagulation (do not offer aspirin instead)
1 = Medium stroke risk (1.3% per annum) = male: OAC if low bleed risk; female: no OAC
≥2 = High risk (>2.2% per annum) = oral anticoagulation recommended

Bleeding risk: **HAS-BLED** or **ORBIT** (NICE recommended)

H	Hypertension = 1		O	Older >75 = 1
A	Abnormal renal/ liver function = 1 for each		R	Reduced Hb (F<12; M<13) = 2
S	Stroke = 1		B	Bleeding = 2
B	Bleeding = 1		I	Insufficient kidney (eGFR <60) = 1
L	Labile INR = 1		T	Treated with antiplatelet = 1
E	Elderly = 1			
D	Drugs (NSAIDs) and alcohol = 1 for each			

≥3 = high risk (avoid oral anticoagulation); >3 = high risk.
Prevalence: 8% of >80-year-olds have AF; 1 in 3 lifetime risk of AF

Hypertension
This 37-year-old female patient presented with intermittent headaches for the past three months. Her blood pressure is elevated. I would be grateful for your opinion.

History
- Duration of symptoms, nature of headache
- Past history of hypertension: previous blood pressure readings (e.g. employment medical, with prescription of oral contraceptive pill, during pregnancy), compliance with therapy
- Other medical history: renal disease, cardiovascular or peripheral vascular disease or risk factors (smoking, diabetes), thyroid disease
- Associated symptoms: chest pain, weakness, abdominal/flank pain; polyuria and muscle cramps (Conn's)
- Drug history (prescribed and illicit – cocaine/amphetamine), alcohol/salt consumption
- Visual disturbance (in accelerated-phase hypertension)
- Paroxysmal symptoms: headache, sweating, palpitations, anxiety (phaeochromocytoma)
- Check if pregnant

Examination
- Appearance: body habitus: obese, Cushingoid, acromegalic
- Radial pulse (SR/AF), radio-radial and radio-femoral delay (coarctation)
- Check the blood pressure yourself, with a manual sphygmomanometer, in both arms – R>L difference >20/10 mm Hg (coarctation, dissection, PVD)
- **Cardiovascular:** heaving, pressure-loaded apex; auscultation: ejection click and ESM (bicuspid AV) associated with coarctation; systolic murmur loudest left infraclavicular; signs of heart failure
- **Renal:** renal bruit(s) – RAS, enlarged ballotable kidney – polycystic kidney disease, current renal replacement therapy (dialysis/transplant), ask to dip the urine
- **Neurological:** visual fields and acuity, focal neurology
- **Fundoscopy:** hypertensive retinopathy

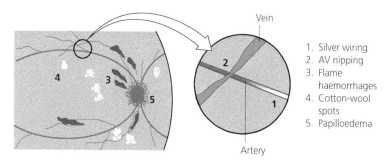

1. Silver wiring
2. AV nipping
3. Flame haemorrhages
4. Cotton-wool spots
5. Papilloedema

GRADES OF HYPERTENSIVE RETINOPATHY
- Grade 1: silver wiring (increased reflectance from thickened arterioles)
- Grade 2: plus arteriovenous nipping (narrowing of veins as arterioles cross them)
- Grade 3: plus cotton-wool spots and flame haemorrhages
- Grade 4: plus papilloedema
- There may also be hard exudates (macular star)

Discussion

CAUSES OF HYPERTENSION

- Essential (94%: associated with age, obesity, salt and alcohol)
- Renal (4%: underlying CKD secondary to glomerulonephritis, ADPKD, renovascular disease)
- Endocrine (1%: Conn's, Cushing's, acromegaly or phaeochromocytoma)
- Aortic coarctation
- Pre-eclampsia: pregnancy

INVESTIGATION

- Evidence of end-organ damage: fundoscopy, LVH on ECG, renal impairment, cardiac failure on CXR, echo
- Exclude underlying cause:
  - Urine pregnancy test (where appropriate!)
  - Urinalysis (and urine ACR)
  - U&Es – low K+, high bicarbonate (Conn's)
  - Consider secondary screen: aldosterone/renin ratio (ARR) – high ARR (>30): Conn's; low ARR due to high renin: secondary e.g., RAS or LVF); plasma and/or urinary metanephrines (phaeo) – if positive consider abdominal CT +/- MRI, MIBG, scintigraphy, FDG-PET: adrenal/ paraganglioma tumour

DIAGNOSIS

- **British Hypertension Society guidelines:**
  - If clinic BP >140/90 mm Hg (measured twice – use lowest); use 24 h ABPM or HBPM to confirm diagnosis (average of daytime values)
  - **Definitions:**
    - **Stage 1 hypertension:** clinic BP ≥140/90 mm Hg or ABPM daytime average ≥135/85 mm Hg
    - **Stage 2 hypertension:** clinic BP ≥160/100 mm Hg or ABPM daytime average ≥150/95 mm Hg
    - **Stage 3/severe hypertension:** clinic SBP ≥180 mm Hg or DBP ≥120 mm Hg
  - Treat if stage 1 hypertension and evidence of end-organ damage, ischaemic heart disease, diabetes, CKD or 10-year cardiovascular risk ≥10%
  - Treat all with stage 2 hypertension
- Arrange same-day admission if severe hypertension and grade 3 or 4 retinopathy (or other concerns, e.g. new renal impairment)

TREATMENT

- Lifestyle modification (lose weight, increase exercise, salt restriction, reduce alcohol, stop smoking)
- Initial treatment:
  - ACE inhibitor or ARB
  - Aged >55 years or Afro-Caribbean ethnicity: ARB/CCB or thiazide-like diuretic
  - Titrate dose to maximum tolerated
- Then add CCB or thiazide-like diuretic (if evidence of CCF use diuretic)
- Then ACE inhibitor/ARB + CCB + thiazide-like diuretic
- Consider adding spironolactone, β-blocker, α-blocker or seeking specialist opinion
- Medications can affect interpretation of renin : aldosterone
- BP target <140/90 mm Hg
  - <150/90 mm Hg if >80 years
  - <130/80 mm Hg if evidence of ACR >70 mg/mmol
  - Lower targets are not recommended for those at higher risk, e.g. AAA or previous CVA
- Consider other cardiovascular risk modification: statin and possibly aspirin (if evidence of CAD/CVA)

- Medical emergency
- **Treatment:**
  - Grade III and IV retinopathy and severe hypertension:
    - Bed rest, oral anti-hypertensives (long-acting CCB) and non-invasive blood pressure monitoring, aiming for gradual reduction in blood pressure
  - Plus encephalopathy/stroke/MI/left ventricular failure/aortic dissection/aneurysm:
    - Parenteral opiate (pain relief); venodilators, e.g. nitroglycerin plus β-blocker, e.g. labetolol (also α-blocker; acute aortic syndromes and phaeo) and invasive blood pressure monitoring
    - Over-rapid fall in blood pressure can lead to 'watershed' cerebral and retinal infarction
    - β-Blocker without α-blocker can precipitate hypertensive crisis in phaeo due to unopposed α-vasoconstriction; perioperative α- and β-blocker advised

- Inherited tumours: 1 in 30,000, autosomal dominant, *RET* gene, 5% de novo mutation
- Classical (MEN 2A):
  - Medullary thyroid cancer (98%)
  - Pheochromocytoma (50%)
  - Parathyroid tumours (5%)

Optic disc swelling

Blurring of disc margins/elevation of disc/loss of venous pulsation/venous engorgement

CAUSES

- **Papilloedema:** raised intracranial pressure from space-occupying lesion, benign intracranial hypertension and cavernous sinus thrombosis – normal visual acuity, enlarged blind spot, usually bilateral
- **Papillitis/optic neuritis:** multiple sclerosis – reduced visual acuity, central scotoma, pain on eye movements, usually unilateral
- **Accelerated phase hypertension:** with hypertensive retinopathy
- **Central retinal vein occlusion:** with large number of haemorrhages, bilateral
- **Anterior ischaemic optic neuropathy:** pale disc, reduced colour vision/loss of vision; arteritic – associated with pain on chewing and scalp tenderness (urgent steroid needed), non-arteritic – painless visual loss

---

Eisenmenger's syndrome
This 37-year-old female patient has noticed worsening breathlessness and blue fingers.

History
- Worsening dyspnoea, peripheral oedema, syncope, palpitations, haemoptysis
- PMH: congenital heart disease
- Explore family planning – pregnancy contraindicated in severe PAH
- Dentition – risk of endocarditis

Complications
- Chronic hypoxaemia causes polycythaemia/viscosity symptoms – dizziness, headache, visual problems, ischaemic skin ulceration, angina, MI, HF and stroke
- Iron deficiency due to polycythaemia
- Gall stones (pigmented, bilirubin), gout and renal stones (urate) due to high RBC turnover
- Paradoxical emboli – stroke

Differential diagnosis
- Other causes of PH, e.g. rheumatological, autoimmune (mixed connective tissue disease, SLE, systemic sclerosis), infectious (Hep B, C, HIV)

Examination
- Central **cyanosis**, **digital clubbing** (toes more than fingers in PDA distal to left subclavian artery), precordium scars, **right parasternal heave**, **loud P2**, murmur (shunt murmur may be absent as right and left chamber pressures similar but **TR** common), right heart failure – high JVP, ascites, hepatomegaly, SOA

Discussion
PATHOPHYSIOLOGY
- Large, often congenital LTR shunts, e.g. ASD, VSD, AVSD, PDA, unrepaired ToF
- Permanent pulmonary vascular changes (vascular smooth muscle proliferation, in situ thrombosis and lumen obliteration), PAH and elevated PVR
- Reverses the shunt direction to RTL causing cyanosis

INVESTIGATION
- CXR (pulmonary vascular pruning, large PA, cardiomegaly), ECG (right heart strain pattern), FBC (polycythaemia), iron studies, BNP
- Lung function tests, CTPA, echo and right heart catheterization

TREATMENT
Medical
- Pulmonary vasodilator therapy, e.g. ERA, PDE5 inhibitor, epoprostenol
- Anticoagulation
- Symptomatic: iron supplementation, allopurinol, diuretic, anti-arrhythmic, oxygen (if hypoxaemia responsive)
- Supportive: contraception (pregnancy contraindicated), avoidance of extreme heat/dehydration (hypotension) and isometric exercise, immunizations, avoidance of relative anaemia
- **Surgical**
  - Correction of shunt is generally contraindicated as RTL shunt prevents worsening PVR and maintains systemic blood flow/O_2 delivery despite hypoxaemia
  - Heart–lung transplantation

PROGNOSIS
- 50% mortality at 1 year

Ataxia

This 46-year-old female patient has been feeling unsteady, with difficulty walking, and has noticed her speech is slurred. She appears to have an abnormal gait. I would be grateful for your urgent assessment.

- **Diagnosis:** multiple sclerosis
- **Differential diagnosis:** vestibular ataxia, stroke, drug/alcohol, Friedreich's ataxia

History

- **Ataxic** – patients often report feeling as though they are drunk
- Associated symptoms – speech, vision (unilateral loss of sight, painful – **optic neuritis**)
- Temporal assessment – **relapsing/remitting** nature of symptoms, separated in time and location, in a young adult is virtually diagnostic of **multiple sclerosis**
- Associated symptoms: lightning pain down back on neck flexion (Lhermitte's sign), depression/euphoria, autonomic: bladder/bowel/impotence
- **Triggers:** presence of Uthoff's phenomenon (worsening of symptoms by heat or exercise)
- **Differential diagnoses:**
  - Risk factors for stroke (diabetes and hypertension)
  - Early-morning headaches/nausea (posterior fossa SOL)
  - Hearing loss/tinnitus/nausea/vomiting/vertigo – feeling of motion in a still environment (vestibular)
  - Previous head/neck injury (vertebral artery dissection)
  - Alcohol history, drug history (phenytoin), diet (vitamin B_{12} deficiency)
  - Family history – Friedreich's ataxia; Wilson's disease
- Ask about activities of daily living, employment (occupational exposure to toxins – mercury)

Examination, investigation and management

- See cerebellar syndrome, multiple sclerosis and Friedreich's ataxia in Neurology
- Grade functional disability, disease impact and risk, e.g. walking – falls; and fine motor skills – dressing/writing/working

Discussion

- **Vestibular ataxia** invariably associated with vertigo and nystagmus and hearing problems in the affected ear. The fast phase of nystagmus is away from the affected ear
- Cause: labyrinthitis/vestibular neuritis due to a viral illness
- Benign self-limiting condition than can take weeks–months to resolve
- **Wilson's disease** is an autosomal recessive condition caused by copper deposition predominantly in liver (jaundice/ascites), brain (neurocognitive including ataxia) and eye (Kayser–Fleischer rings); low ceruloplasmin is often present

Headache

This 27-year-old female university student attended the GP surgery this morning complaining of a severe headache. She has photophobia and has been vomiting. Please could you urgently assess her.

- **Diagnosis:** migrainous headache
- **Differential diagnosis:** bacterial meningitis (most important to exclude), subarachnoid haemorrhage

History
- Headaches such as migraine, tension headache or cluster headache are **primary** headaches
- History and neurological examination are the key to distinguishing them from **secondary** headaches (e.g. subarachnoid haemorrhage, meningitis, temporal arteritis)

SYMPTOMS CONSISTENT WITH MENINGITIS
- **Meningism:** neck stiffness, headache and photophobia
- Nausea and vomiting
- Focal neurological deficit, **constitutional symptoms** of infection, e.g. fever, rash
- Risk factors: immunosuppressed, **close meningitis contact** and foreign travel

SYMPTOMS SUGGESTIVE OF SUBARACHNOID HAEMORRHAGE
- Sudden onset, severe **'thunderclap' headache** (maximum intensity within 5 min) – SAH is present in about 20% of patients with thunderclap headache
- May be preceded by 'warning' sentinel headaches (but only in about 6%)
- May be associated with collapse at the time of headache
- Risk factors – **hypertension**, ask about family history (ADPKD), smoking, bleeding disorders/medications

PRIMARY HEADACHE DIFFERENTIAL DIAGNOSIS
- **Migrainous headache:**
  ○ Mnemonic **POUND**ing headache (**P**ulsating, duration of 4–72 h**O**urs, **U**nilateral, **N**ausea, **D**isabling)
  ○ **Triggers:** stress, tiredness, chocolate and red wine
  ○ Often exacerbated by head movement and mild exertion
  ○ **Recurrent and frequent:** 1–2 attacks per month for a few months (typical for primary)
  ○ May be associated photophobia, phonophobia (aggravated by loud noises), nausea and vomiting
  ○ May have preceding **aura**, e.g. scintillating scotoma, visual fortification spectra, sensory symptoms, speech disturbance and focal neurological deficits in 30%
  ○ Autonomic features may occur
- Other common primary headache disorders:
  ○ **Tension headache:**
    ○ Bilateral, pressing, moderate but not disabling
    ○ Attacks last hours–days
    ○ Not aggravated by normal activity
  ○ **Cluster headache:**
    ○ Unilateral only
    ○ Very severe, last 15 min to a few hours, frequent attacks each day, may be worse at night
    ○ Patient is restless and/or agitated
    ○ More common in men than women
    ○ There may be autonomic features ipsilateral to the headache: conjunctival injection, lacrimation, nasal congestion, rhinorrhoea

- **Trigeminal neuralgia:**
  - Paroxysms of severe, stabbing pain in the trigeminal nerve distribution (usually maxillary or mandibular).
  - May be triggered – e.g. touching, shaving
- **Medication overuse headache:**
  - Patients with an episodic headache disorder using opiates (including codeine ± paracetamol), triptans, ergotamine for 10 or more days/month for >3 months, converting this into a chronic headache disorder

TREATMENT CONSIDERATIONS

- Allergies to penicillin
- Always check if female patients may be pregnant

Examination

LOOK FOR MENINGISM

- Neck stiffness
- Photophobia on fundoscopy
- **Kernig's sign:** hip flexion and knee: flexion → extension is painful and resisted (avoid causing pain in the exam!)
- Fever

LOOK FOR A RASH

- Meningococcal meningitis: **petechial/purpura rash** indicates associated septicaemia (does not blanch on compressing)

BRIEF NEUROLOGICAL EXAMINATION

- You should perform a brief but thorough neurological examination (see Neurology)
- You are seeking to identify focal neurological signs
- Don't forget to perform fundoscopy and ask the patient to walk
- **Cerebral abscess:**
  - **Localizing signs:** upper limb: pronator drift; lower limb: extensor plantar; cranial nerve palsy
- Cerebral oedema/increasing intracranial pressure (unlikely in the exam):
  - Reduced Glasgow Coma Scale score, unilateral dilated pupil (third nerve palsy) and papilloedema

HAEMODYNAMIC STABILITY

- Septic shock: pulse and BP

Discussion

INVESTIGATION

- **Meningitis:**
  - Blood culture
  - **Lumbar puncture:**
    - Will need **head CT first** to exclude raised intracranial pressure if localizing signs or altered conscious state
  - Send CSF sample for MC + S, glucose (with blood glucose) and protein:
    - Bacterial: low glucose, high protein, neutrophils and gram + cocci
    - Viral: normal glucose and protein, mononuclear cells
- **SAH:**
  - **Urgent CT head**
    - Approximately 99% sensitive for SAH if performed <6 h of headache onset
  - If CT normal then LP >12 h of headache onset (bilirubin/xanthochromia, which takes time to form in the CSF) as well as standard protein/glucose/microscopy
    - Differentiate bloody tap from subarachnoid haemorrhage by assessing xanthochromia (bilirubin from degraded RBCs turn CSF yellow)

TREATMENT

Meningitis:
- o Do not delay antibiotics:
  - o Penicillin: high dose, intravenous immediately if diagnosis is suspected
- o Meningitis is a notifiable disease:
  - o Treat close contacts
- **SAH:**
  - o Urgent neurosurgical referral, nimodipine to reduce vasospasm
- **Migraine:**
  - o Acute treatments – aspirin (600–900 mg), NSAIDs, antiemetics, triptans
  - o Preventative treatments – consider what best suits the patient, options include amitriptyline, propranolol, candesartan, topiramate and monoclonal antibodies against CGRP (calcitonin gene-related peptide)
- **Tension headache:**
  - o Simple analgesics (aspirin, paracetamol)
- **Cluster headaches:**
  - o Oxygen and triptans for acute attacks
  - o Prevention – verapamil, short courses of oral steroids
- Signpost the patient towards useful information – the British Association for the Study of Headache (BASH) website is excellent, with clear guidelines: https://bash.org.uk

---

Causes of thunderclap headache
- SAH
- Meningitis
- Intracranial haemorrhage
- Cerebral venous sinus thrombosis
- Malignant hypertension

Altered conscious state
This 48-year-old male patient with diabetes mellitus has been found drowsy and confused.

- **Diagnosis:** diabetic ketoacidosis
- **Differential diagnosis:** meningitis and alcohol/drug intoxication

History
SYMPTOMS (FROM A WITNESS/RELATIVE)
- **Polyuria and polydipsia**
- Preceding acute illness/fever
- Recent high glucometer readings/increased insulin requirement
- Associated symptoms: nausea, sweating and breathlessness

RISK FACTORS FOR DIABETIC KETOACIDOSIS
- Poor **compliance** with insulin: young, change in social circumstances

DIFFERENTIAL DIAGNOSIS
- Smelling of alcohol (take care not ketotic), history of drug abuse
- Alcohol and drug history

Examination
CONFIRMATION OF DIAGNOSIS
- Determine Glasgow Coma Scale score
- Breath: **'pear-drops'** (ketones)
- Hyperventilation or Kussmaul's breathing: metabolic acidosis
- Medic alert bracelet/finger prick marks: diabetes

PRECIPITATING FACTORS
- **4 Is** – **I**nsulin forgotten, **I**nfection, **I**nfarction and **I**njury

COMPLICATIONS
- Retina: diabetic changes, papilloedema
- Pulse and BP: haemodynamic compromise
- Auscultate chest: aspiration pneumonia
- Gastroparesis due to diabetic autonomic neuropathy

Discussion
INVESTIGATIONS
- Finger prick glucometer
- Urine dipstick and finger prick for ketones
- ABG:
  - Metabolic acidosis with respiratory compensation ($\downarrow PaCO_2$)
  - Monitor response to treatment with venous HCO_3-
- FBC, U&E, LFT and glucose
- ECG (silent MI)
- Blood and urine cultures (sepsis)
- CXR (pneumonia or aspiration)

TREATMENT
- ABC:
  - May require intubation and ITU support
- Fluid resuscitation: crystalloid
  - Consider K^+ supplementation
- IV insulin sliding scale
- Consider:
  - NG tube to prevent aspiration
  - SC heparin for VTE prophylaxis
  - Antibiotics for infection

Syncope

Please evaluate this 75-year-old female patient who blacked out at the dinner table without warning.

Differential diagnosis
- **Cardiac:** brady- or tachycardia; brady: post-op SAVR or TAVI, Lyme, sarcoid, obstructive cardiac lesion: AS, MS, HOCM; PH
- **Neurological:** epilepsy, vertebrobasilar insufficiency, EtOH, diabetes
- **Orthostatic (postural) hypotension:** vasodilator drugs
- **Vasovagal (neurocardiogenic):** stress, cough, micturition, defecation
- **Psychogenic non-epileptic spells:** psychiatric 'pseudo-seizures'

History
- Description of the syncopal episode – often perplexed: 'found myself on the floor' plus significant injury then likely syncope
  - **Provocation:** micturition, cough or stressful situation (vasovagal), flashing lights, fever, hypoglycaemia (neuro)
  - **Posture:** sitting/lying (cardiac) or standing (orthostatic), sudden head turning (vertebrobasilar)
  - **Prodrome:** light-headed, dizziness, tunnel vision, sweaty, tinnitus (vasovagal/orthostatic); no warning (cardiac); mood change, déjà vu, anxiety, aura: olfactory, visual obscuration, paraesthesia (neuro)
  - **Associated symptoms:** palpitations and chest pain (cardiac); headache, tongue biting and incontinence (neuro)
  - Duration (transient, <5 min) and frequency
  - **Recovery:** immediate (cardiac) or prolonged confused state and amnesia (>5 min) (neuro), red/flushed face (cardiac)
  - Injury (neuro or cardiac)
  - **Eyewitness account** is very useful
- Past medical history of syncope/presyncope, cardiac disease (MI) or neurological conditions (stroke, head injury)
- Other diagnoses: sarcoidosis and Lyme disease (tick bites) cause heart block, brain SOL (early-morning headache) causes seizures, diabetes (hypoglycaemic seizure)
- Medications that may cause hypotension, compliance
- **Alcohol** (withdrawal can cause seizures)
- Family history of epilepsy
- Social impact of diagnosis – driving, work; general safety – bathing alone

Examination
FOCUSED CARDIOLOGY EXAMINATION
- Pulse and blood pressure (lying and standing), **postural drop:** >20/10 mm Hg difference
- Auscultation: **obstructive valvular pathology**, e.g. AS or MS, or signs of PH (loud P_2 and left parasternal heave)
- **Pacemaker or ICD** scars

FOCUSED NEUROLOGICAL EXAMINATION
- Fundoscopy
- Pronator drift
- Upper-limb tone and reflexes
- Parkinson's signs

OTHER
- Signs of chronic liver disease, diabetes

Discussion

INVESTIGATION

- **12-lead ECG**, Holter monitor, implantable loop recorder, electrophysiology study, ETT and **echo** if cardiac cause suspected
- Tilt table test if orthostatic hypotension suspected
- **EEG** and/or **CT MRI brain** if a neurological cause is suspected

MANAGEMENT

- **Cardiac:** pacemaker, ICD, revascularization and valvular surgery
- **Vasovagal:** education on avoidance, isotonic muscle contraction
- **Orthostatic hypotension:** salt and water replacement, support stockings, medication review, occasionally synthetic mineralocorticoid fludrocortisone, α-agonist midodrine are helpful
- **Neurological:** anticonvulsants – counsel about side effects, pregnancy (teratogenic, folic acid) and contraception (may alter effectiveness of OCP); stereotactic brain stimulation/surgery; avoid triggers: alcohol, sleep, compliance, medic alert bracelet, personal safety

SEIZURES

- **Generalized** (absence; tonic–clonic; atonic – altered conscious state) or **partial (simple** – patient aware, may give clue to brain pathology; **complex** – staring blankly, daydreaming, commonest; may have secondary generalization)
- **Epilepsy:** two or more unprovoked seizures >24 h apart
- Two-thirds of patients with epilepsy no cause found
- See Epilepsy in Communication section

MULTISYSTEM ATROPHY (MSA):

- Tremor, rigidity, bradykinesia – Parkinson's (MSA-P)
- Cerebellar ataxia (MSA-C) and autonomic dysfunction: **orthostatic hypotension** causing collapse, impotence, urinary retention/incontinence, dry mouth, hoarse voice (vocal cord palsy), swallow problems

LYME DISEASE

- Deer tick bite – *Borrelia burgdorferi*
- Erythema migrans – 'bullseye' spreading from site of bite, fever, headache, fatigue, joint pain, rarely facial palsy
- Lyme carditis – 1 in 100 cases: atrioventricular heart block causing syncope, SOB and chest pain
- Diagnosis: detect antibody a few weeks after infection
- Treatment antibiotics, TPW – usually full recovery within 1–6 weeks

DVLA

- **Group 1 licence: car/motorbike:**
  ○ Check the 3 Ps: **p**rovocation/**p**rodrome/**p**ostural – if all present then likely benign and can continue driving
  ○ Solitary with no clear cause – 6-month ban; clear cause that has been treated – resume driving after 4 weeks
  ○ Recurrent syncope due to seizures – must be fit free for 1 year to drive

Worsening mobility
Please can you assess this 87-year-old male who has worsening mobility.

- **Diagnosis:** UTI
- **Differential diagnosis:** drug side effects, pneumonia, cerebrovascular disease, Parkinson's

History
WHAT HAS HAPPENED TO HIS MOBILITY?
- Gradual or stepwise decline
- Time course (days/weeks/months)
- How far can he walk now and with what aids?
- How far could he walk when he was 'well' and how long ago was this?
- History of falls

PRECIPITANT
- Infection:
  - Urinary symptoms: **dysuria, frequency and incontinence**
  - Pneumonia: cough and breathlessness
- Drug changes recently: benzodiazepines (sleepiness), diuretics and BP medication (postural hypotension), antipsychotic (extrapyramidal side effects), steroids (proximal myopathy), anti-parkinsonian drug changes, hypoglycaemic agents
- Systemic enquiry: sites of pain

SIGNIFICANT MEDICAL HISTORY
- Previous related pathology – stroke, Parkinson's disease, etc.
- Diabetes, hypertension, ischaemic heart disease, prostatism (sources of polypharmacy)
- Recent hospital stays (sources of deconditioning)
- Cognition
- Weight loss

SOCIAL HISTORY
- Independence → dependence
- Mobility issues related to Parkinsonism, stroke etc.
- Unaided → stick → frame
- Recent falls
- **Social circumstances:**
  - Current accommodation and type (house, flat)
  - Who he lives with (alone/spouse/daughter and extended family)
  - Current care needs – and are they being met?
  - Who are the carers – family, private or state-funded?

LEGAL ASPECTS
- Advanced directives or living wills
- Power of attorney
- DNAR and other treatments

Examination
- A lot of information can be obtained by asking the patient to **stand and walk** unaided (ensure patient safety):
  - Proximal lower-limb motor strength: rising from a chair
  - Gait: wide-based/ataxic (cerebellar), hemiplegic (stroke) and shuffling (Parkinson's syndrome)
  - Complete a focused neurological examination – guided by history

- **Romberg's test:**
  - Positive if patient stumbles forward on closing their eyes (protect the patient from falling when assessing this), indicating a problem with proprioception (sensory nerves and dorsal columns)
  - Balance requires sensory input from at least two of the following three inputs: vision, the vestibular apparatus and proprioception. If proprioception is impaired and vision removed you are reliant on the vestibular system alone, which is not enough
- **Postural dizziness:**
  - Assess lying and standing BP (or at least state that you would – there is unlikely to be time in the exam)
  - >20 mm Hg drop in systolic BP from lying to standing is significant (but should be recorded on standing, and for the next 3 min while upright)
- Examine for signs of infection – guided by history

Discussion

INVESTIGATIONS
- **Septic screen:** urine culture, blood cultures and CXR
- Remember – don't ask for urinalysis (to look for infection) in those aged >65 years (high false-positive rate)
- Baseline investigations: FBC (anaemia, infection), U&E (hyponatraemia, AKI), CRP, calcium
- ECG ('silent' MI)

MANAGEMENT
- Treat reversible causes: antibiotics as indicated, **avoid polypharmacy** (stop unnecessary medications)
- **MDT approach:** nurse, social worker, occupational therapy and physiotherapy
  - Mobility aids
  - Reducing falls risk
  - Rehabilitation
  - **Care package:** home improvements or residential care
- Ceiling of care with patient and family
  - ReSPECT form – **resuscitation decision**

Fall and a fragility fracture

This 84-year-old female has had a mechanical fall and Colles fracture. Please assess her.

- **Diagnosis:** osteoporosis
- **Differential diagnosis:** bone metastasis, secondary hyperparathyroidism (CKD)

History

- Confirm **mechanical fall** – patients often remember how they fell and broke their fall (with outstretched arm), describing 'losing balance', 'trip', 'legs give way', rather than dizziness, altered consciousness seen with syncope
- **Frailty assessment** (e.g. Rockwood Frailty scale): recent hospitalization, low physical activity, incontinence, unintentional weight loss, self-reported exhaustion, help with ADLs
- Mechanical falls risk assessment: frailty, previous fall, poor eyesight, reduced mobility and cognition, polypharmacy causing postural hypotension, poor footwear, inappropriate housing (stairs/trip hazards)
- **Osteoporotic risk assessment** (fragility fracture – hip, wrist, vertebral):
  - Gynaecological: early menopause, hysterectomy and BSO <45 years old, HRT
  - Drug history: corticosteroid
  - Social history: smoking, alcohol misuse
  - Family history of osteoporosis or hip fracture
- **Associated diagnoses:** hyperthyroidism, pituitary gland – hypogonadism, breast (or prostate in men) cancer treatments (oestrogen or testosterone antagonists), hyperparathyroidism, malabsorption calcium and vit D (coeliac), RA, low BMI

Examination

GENERAL
- 'Get up and go' from a chair – assesses strength, gait, balance and mobility (be sure it is safe to do so)
- Lymphadenopathy, hepatomegaly, masses, cachexia (malignancy)

CARDIOVASCULAR
- Postural hypotension, aortic valve stenosis

NEUROLOGICAL
- Assess for signs of Parkinson's, cerebellar signs, focal neurology, lower-limb muscle strength, proprioception, vision, cognitive assessment

Discussion

INVESTIGATION
- Bloods: FBC (iron deficiency); U&E, Cr (CKD), LFT, TFT; Ca++, PTH; serum protein electrophoresis for paraprotein/immunoglobulins (multiple myeloma); tTG-IgA (coeliac)
- **DXA scan** to assess bone mineral density: T-score <–2.5
- If fall and altered conscious state/confusion consider CT head: subdural haematoma, especially in atrophic brain

MANAGEMENT
- Multidisciplinary approach: occupational therapy, physiotherapy, social worker, dietician
- **Lifestyle:**
  - Education, exercise programmes – strength exercises
  - Hip protectors, visual aids
  - Diet: healthy weight, high protein, calcium rich
- **Medical:**
  - Rationalize medication and avoid polypharmacy, psychotropics, hypotensive medication
  - Vitamin D_3 and calcium supplementation
  - HRT and bisphosphonates – review every 3–5 years

Dyspnoea – asthma
Please assess this young female with sudden-onset breathlessness.

- **Diagnosis:** asthma
- **Differential diagnosis:** PE, pneumothorax, anaemia, respiratory tract infection

History
ASTHMA
- **Sudden-onset wheeze**, shortness of breath and cough (non-productive)
- Triggers
  - **Allergy:**
    - Pets, food, dust and pollen
    - Atopic: allergic rhinitis and eczema
    - Anaphylaxis
    - Allergy-testing clinic
  - Upper respiratory tract infection: sore throat, fever, etc.
- **Severity:**
  - Previous hospital admissions
  - ITU admissions and intubation
- **Peak expiratory flow rate (PEFR):** best, normal and current
- Vaccination status: Covid-19 and influenza, particularly if infection is trigger
- Drug history:
  - Compliance with preventor medication
  - Inhaler technique
  - EpiPen®

DIFFERENTIAL DIAGNOSIS
- Pneumothorax:
  - Spontaneous in asthmatics or tall, thin individuals
  - Permanent pacemaker or central line
- Symptoms and risk factors for DVT causing PE

Examination
SEVERITY (DOES THIS PATIENT NEED ITU?)
- Conscious level
- Respiratory rate:
  - **Count 1–10:** how far do they get on one breath?
- Pulse and blood pressure
- **Check PEFR** (best of three)

RESPIRATORY
- **Asthma:** expansion and percussion note increased bilaterally due to lung hyper-expansion, polyphonic wheeze (silent chest is a sign of severity)
- **Anaphylaxis:** stridor, angioedema and tongue swelling
- **Pneumothorax:** unilateral reduced expansion and breath sounds and increased resonance on percussion; tracheal and/or apex beat deviation away (tension pneumothorax)

OTHER
- Urticaria (anaphylaxis)
- Calf swelling (DVT → PE)
- Fever (LRTI)
- Pale (anaemia)

Discussion

INVESTIGATIONS

- Arterial blood gas:
  - Hypoxaemia
  - **Normal or rising PaCO$_2$** suggests a tiring patient requiring respiratory support (should have a respiratory alkalosis if coping)
- CXR in exhalation (pneumothorax), consolidation (pneumonia)
- CTPA (PE)

TREATMENT

- Asthma:
  - Bronchodilators and steroids (not routine antibiotics as often viral)
  - Asthma specialist nurse:
    - Inhaler technique
    - Allergy clinic
- Pneumothorax:
  - Needle aspiration or chest drain
  - May need talc or surgical pleurodesis if it is recurrent

Grading severity of acute asthma exacerbation

Moderate	• PEFR 50–75% of best or predicted • None of the features below
Severe	Any one of: • PEFR 33–50% of best or predicted • Respiratory rate ≥25/min • Heart rate ≥110/min • Inability to complete sentences in one breath
Life-threatening	Any one of: • PERF <33% of best or predicted • Altered conscious level, exhaustion, arrhythmia, hypotension, silent chest, cyanosis, poor respiratory effort • SpO$_2$ <92% • PaO$_2$ <8 kPa • 'Normal' PaCO$_2$ (4.6–6.0 kPa)

With permission of British Thoracic Society.

CRITERIA FOR SAFE DISCHARGE

- Clinical signs suitable for home management
- PEFR >75% best or predicted
- Check inhaler technique and ability to record PEFR
- Written asthma management plan
- Follow-up arranged with patient's GP/asthma nurse within two working days
- Hospital follow-up in one month (respiratory physician or asthma specialist nurse)

Dyspnoea – acute pulmonary embolus

Please assess this 33-year-old female teacher who has experienced pleuritic chest pain and dyspnoea for the last three days.

History
- What were they doing when the pain started?
- Speed of onset (seconds–minutes)?
- Nature of the pain – **pleuritic**? Worse when breathing in, coughing?
- **Dyspnoea** – and how severe (on exertion/at rest)?
- Cough ± **haemoptysis**
- Calf/thigh pain and/or swelling
- Pre-syncopal symptoms
- Previous VTE
- **Family history**
- Risk factors for VTE (**Wells' criteria**):
    - Immobility for ≥3 days or surgery within the previous 3 weeks
    - Known malignancy
    - Combined oral contraceptive pill
    - Current or recent pregnancy
    - Long-distance travel (>4 h – flight/coach/car journey where mobility is restricted)
    - Smoking
- Ask about other medical conditions and current medication

Examination
- General observations – HR, RR, BP
- Cervical lymphadenopathy (malignancy)
- Respiratory exam – rub, crepitations (differential diagnosis – pleural effusion, LRTI)
- CVS – loud P_2, raised JVP
- Focused abdominal exam – masses, hepatomegaly
- Lower limbs – signs of DVT (swelling and tenderness, tenderness along deep veins)

Discussion
INVESTIGATION
- Determined by pre-test probability of PE e.g., using Wells' criteria
    - **Low-intermediate pre-test probability: D-dimer level** (sensitive but not specific – negative = rule out)
        - Consider – FBC, CRP, U&E for other diagnoses
        - Clotting profile
        - Urine pregnancy test
        - ECG
        - CXR
    - **High pre-test probability or positive D-dimer** – proceed to imaging with **CTPA or ventilation/perfusion (VQ)** (specific – positive = rule in) depending on local protocols, need to assess other diagnoses
        - Consider Doppler ultrasound of the affected lower limb if there are clear signs of a DVT

TREATMENT
- **Anticoagulation** may already have started in the community
- Don't delay anticoagulation while awaiting imaging – often anticoagulation is started and low-risk patients are discharged to return for next-day imaging
- Anticoagulation options:
    - DOAC – rivaroxaban or apixaban
    - Treatment-dose low molecular weight heparin

- ○ Warfarin
- ○ Counsel the patient about the benefits of anticoagulation, when to seek medical help, and offer them written advice
- ○ Duration of treatment – at least three months (longer if unprovoked)
- Contraindications to anticoagulation – consider IVC filter
- Thrombectomy, ultrasonic dissolution, local lytic for sub-massive PE with right heart strain
- Systemic thrombolytic therapy for massive life-threatening PE

FURTHER INVESTIGATIONS
- None needed if clearly provoked first PE (e.g. recent surgery, immobility)
- If unprovoked and/or recurrent PE:
  - ○ Review baseline bloods, check calcium and LFT
  - ○ Exclude nephrotic syndrome (urine dip and serum albumin)
  - ○ Examine for possible malignancy (as above)
  - ○ Any further investigation for cancer should be based on history and examination – routine CT screening is not recommended (NICE Guidance 2023)
  - ○ Do not offer routine thrombophilia testing unless first-degree relative with VTE or recurrent VTE – this can be delayed until the planned anticoagulation cessation
- Consider follow-up (hospital/GP) at three months, with BNP, echo, repeat VQ or CTPA, 6MWD, CPET if persistent dyspnoea (chronic thromboembolic pulmonary hypertension – CTEPH)

CTEPH (Group 4 PH)
- Persistent SOB, fatigue, dizziness >3/12 after acute PE despite oral anticoagulation
- Failure to resorb clot – organized into webs, confirmed on CTPA/MRI or VQ
- Pulmonary hypertension (mPAP >20 mm Hg, PCWP <15 mm Hg, PVR >3 WU) and right heart failure
- Treatment – medical: riociguat, continued OAC; interventional: BPA; surgical: PEA

Haemoptysis
Please assess this 74-year-old smoker who complains of a cough with blood-stained sputum for the last three weeks.

- **Diagnosis:** bronchial carcinoma
- **Differential diagnosis:** pulmonary embolus, pneumonia, pulmonary oedema

History
SYMPTOMS SUGGESTIVE OF MALIGNANCY
- Cough: chronicity, mucous colour and **haemoptysis**
- Breathlessness
- Chest pain: pleuritic
- General: **weight loss** (cachexia), bone pain (metastasis) and tiredness (anaemia)
- Rare manifestations of CA bronchus, e.g. paraneoplastic neuropathy
- Abdominal pain: liver metastases or hypercalcaemia
- Headache, new focal neurology: brain metastasis

RISK FACTORS
- **Smoking** history:
  - Calculate number of pack years (20 years' smoking 40 cigarettes/day = 40 pack years)
- Occupation: industrial chemicals, coal dust

DIFFERENTIAL DIAGNOSIS
- Risk factors for DVT/PE
- Past medical history of ischaemic heart disease and HF – frothy, pink sputum.
- Constitutional symptoms for pneumonia: fever and productive cough

Examination
PERIPHERAL STIGMATA OF BRONCHIAL CARCINOMA
- Cachexia
- Nail **clubbing** and tar-stained fingers (smoking)
- Tattoos from previous radiotherapy

RESPIRATORY EXAMINATION
- Cervical lymphadenopathy
- Tracheal deviation: lobar collapse
- Dull percussion note: consolidation and effusion
- Reduced air entry/bronchial breathing

METASTASES
- Craggy hepatomegaly
- Spinal tenderness on percussion with heel of hand
- Focal neurology: cerebral metastases

Discussion
INVESTIGATION
- CXR: mass, pleural effusion and bone erosion
- **CT chest**/staging CT (including lower neck, liver and adrenals)
- CT PET for potentially curative disease
- Bronchoscopy/CT-guided **biopsy**/endobronchial ultrasound (EBUS) ± biopsy or lymph biopsy/excision: tissue diagnosis
- Brain imaging: depends on symptoms and stage of disease

Histology classification:
- o Small cell lung cancer (SCLC) – 10–15% of lung cancers
  - o Usually disseminated at presentation
  - o Older, male smokers
- o Non-small cell lung cancer (NSCLC) – 80–85% of lung cancers
  - o Main subtypes: adenocarcinoma, squamous cell carcinoma, large cell carcinoma
  - o Most common in older smokers or ex-smokers, but adenocarcinoma is the commonest type in non-smokers

- Surgical: lobectomy
- Medical:
  - o Chemotherapy:
    - o Platinum-based chemotherapy for SCLC and NSCLC
    - o Tumour mutation analysis drives choice of systemic anti-cancer therapy for NSCLC, e.g. immune-checkpoint inhibitors
  - o Radiotherapy
  - o Palliative care

Pancoast's tumour
Tumour of the lung apex, may present with:

- Shoulder pain – posterior and sharp
- **Ipsilateral Horner's syndrome**: ptosis, miosis, anhidrosis and enophthalmos (from tumour invasion of the paravertebral sympathetic chain)
- Brachial plexus involvement and neurological signs in the **ipsilateral upper limb – weakness and atrophy in muscles of the hand**
- **Supraclavicular lymphadenopathy**
- Weight loss

Persistent fever
Please assess this young male patient with fever and malaise for the last three months.

- **Diagnosis:** infection (endocarditis)
- **Differential diagnosis:** drug-induced, malignancy (lymphoma), inflammatory disease (SLE, RA), factitious

History
INFECTION
- Associated symptoms: sweating, **rigor,** myalgia, **fatigue** (general); **rash**, headache, photophobia, meningism (meningitis), seizures, confusion, focal weakness (embolic – endocarditis, brain abscess), joint/bone pain (arthralgia/osteomyelitis), abdominal pain (abscess), toothache (dental abscess), dysuria (UTI) or cough (lung abscess/pneumonia)
- **Temporal pattern:**
  ○ Fever at night: malaria
  ○ **Chronic over months:** endocarditis
- Infectious contacts:
  ○ TB, EBV, Covid-19
  ○ Immunization record
  ○ History of blood transfusions – hep B, C, HIV
- PMH:
  ○ **Cardiac problems:** valvular or congenital heart disease
  ○ **Dental problems, invasive procedures** and **antibiotic prophylaxis**
- FH:
  ○ Familial Mediterranean fever – genetic auto-inflammatory disorder: serositis affecting joints, abdomen, chest; may cause amyloidosis
- SH:
  ○ Foreign travel to areas with endemic diseases:
    ○ Malarial regions and compliance with prophylaxis
  ○ Sexual:
    ○ HIV risk – counsel regarding testing
  ○ Pets/animal exposure, e.g. dairy farmer (brucellosis)
  ○ **Drug abuse/homelessness:**
    ○ Infective endocarditis and TB/HIV risk
    ○ Amphetamine use
  ○ Environmental:
    ○ Heatstroke/sunburn
    ○ **Weight loss**
  ○ Psychiatric history/stress (factitious):
    ○ Medical background

DRUG
- After change in medication (drug-induced)
- Malignant hyperpyrexia syndrome:
  ○ Antipsychotic medication
  ○ Associated with muscle pain, rigidity
- Allergies to antibiotic and antibiotic history

MALIGNANCY
- Weight loss
- Lumps: painless lymphadenopathy, bruising (lymphoma and HIV)
- Smoker, breathlessness and chest pain (lung)
- Altered bowel habit (colon)

- Joint or skin problems: SLE, RA, PMR
- Granulomatous disease: Crohn's, sarcoid
- Giant cell arteritis

Examination
PERIPHERAL
- **Temperature >38 °C** (elderly may be normal), flushed, dehydrated – tachycardia, dry mucous membranes
- Look for needle tracks
- **Splinter haemorrhages** (fingers)
- **Roth spots** (fundoscopy)
- **Poor dentition**
- Lymphadenopathy

CARDIOVASCULAR
- **Murmur:** endocarditis

ABDOMINAL EXAMINATION
- Craggy liver or mass (malignancy)
- **Splenomegaly** (infection, inflammatory and malignancy)
- Dip the urine: **haematuria** (endocarditis)

JOINTS, SKIN AND EYES
- Inflammatory conditions – tender scalp absent pulses (temporal arteritis), hot swollen joint, red rash

Discussion
INVESTIGATION
- Septic screen:
  - **Blood culture** including repeated thick and thin film (parasitaemia)
  - Urine and CSF
  - Serology: EBV, CMV, HIV testing (screening – high sensitivity)
  - Molecular PCR: HIV (confirmation – high specificity)
  - Procalcitonin – high specificity for bacterial infection
- **CRP**, ESR, autoantibodies, immunoglobulins (myeloma) and complement levels
- CK (malignant hyperthermia)
- **TTE and TOE:** vegetations, aortic root abscess and myxoma
- US abdomen (masses, collection), venous Doppler (DVT)
- Cross-sectional imaging: **CT chest abdomen pelvis**, MRI, ^{18}F-FDG-PET and white cell scintigraphy for vasculitis, small foci of tumour/infection
- Biopsy – temporal artery, liver, lymph node, bone marrow

MANAGEMENT
- If patient not critically unwell, **avoid early empiric antibiotics** or steroid until identification of the cause
- **Bacterial endocarditis:**
  - Six weeks of intravenous antibiotics
  - Cardiothoracic surgery – valve replacement, particularly if:
    - Large, sessile vegetation >1 cm
    - Embolic phenomena
    - Heart failure
    - Failure to respond to antibiotics

- Consider stopping all drugs and reinstituting them one by one
- Supportive: **pyrolytic**, e.g. paracetamol, ibuprofen, fan, cool sponges; oral and IV **hydration**
- Specific: investigate and treat underlying cause
- Admit the patient and monitor them closely:
  - Fever that resolves during close observation without treatment may be factitious!

Anaemia

This housebound elderly female patient has become more anaemic and is breathless. Please assess her.

- **Diagnosis:** iron deficiency anaemia (dietary)
- **Differential diagnosis:** chronic GI bleeding; coeliac; inherited haemoglobinopathy, e.g. β-thalassaemia trait

History

SYMPTOMS OF ANAEMIA (OFTEN NON-SPECIFIC)
- Tiredness, lethargy and breathlessness
- Angina
- Gastrointestinal
  - ○ Stools: altered bowel habit, foul smelling (**steatorrhoea** – malabsorption, e.g. coeliac), tarry (**malaena** – upper GI bleed)
  - ○ **Weight loss** (malabsorption)
  - ○ Indigestion history, GORD, dysphagia and use of **NSAIDs**
  - ○ **Abdominal pain**/bloating and wheat intolerance (coeliac)
- Previous history
  - ○ Surgery: small bowel resection or **peptic ulcer**
  - ○ Inflammatory bowel disease and polyps
  - ○ **Menstruation:** heavy periods or PV bleeding
- Family history
  - ○ GI malignancy
  - ○ Anaemia: Mediterranean – thalassaemia; Afro-Caribbean – sickle cell
- Travel history
  - ○ Hookworm or tropical sprue
- Dietary history
  - ○ Vegetarian or **vegan**; elderly 'tea and toast' – low dietary iron
- Planning treatment
  - ○ Previous blood transfusions/transfusion reactions

Examination

CONFIRM ANAEMIA
- General pallor
- Pale conjunctivae

DETERMINE CAUSE OF ANAEMIA
- Nails: koilonychia (iron deficiency)
- Mouth: glossitis, angular stomatitis (iron and vitamin B deficiency)
- Sentinel cervical lymph node
- Abdominal mass and hepatomegaly (GI malignancy), epigastric tenderness
- Abdominal scars: small bowel, colon resection
- Offer to perform rectal and vaginal examinations

DETERMINE EFFECT OF ANAEMIA
- Pulse (tachycardiac) and BP: haemodynamic stability; aortic valve flow murmur

DISCUSSION
- Dietary deficiency causing anaemia is a diagnosis of exclusion

COELIAC DISEASE (GLUTEN-SENSITIVE ENTEROPATHY)
- Autoimmune disease causing small bowel villous atrophy and malabsorption
- Anaemia (iron, B_{12}, folate deficiency), dry eyes (vitamin A deficiency), ataxia and neuropathy, dermatitis herpetiformis (itchy blistering rash on extensor surfaces; IgA

deposits in dermis on punch biopsy), osteoporosis (calcium and vit D deficiency), aphthous ulcers, infertility, growth retardation
- Increased risk of small bowel lymphoma, other autoimmune diseases (T1DM, PBC, Hashimoto's thyroiditis)
- Diagnosis (while exposed to gluten): IgA tissue transglutaminase antibody + and total IgA normal, typical histology on duodenal biopsy – villous atrophy
- Treatment: gluten-free diet

INVESTIGATIONS
- **Full blood count** – microcytic anaemia and target cells:
  - **Iron↓, ferritin↓, total iron binding capacity**↑ (folate and vitamin B_{12})
  - Haemoglobin electrophoresis:
    - Thalassaemia and HbE
- Faecal occult blood
- **Endoscopy:** gastroscopy and colonoscopy
- CT abdomen/barium studies

TREATMENT
- Treat the cause
- Dietary advice and **iron supplementation** – oral or intravenous
- Blood transfusion indicated only in extremis (transfusion trigger Hb <70 g/L), but may be higher if patient has comorbidity, e.g. coronary artery disease

---

Osler–Weber–Rendu syndrome (hereditary haemorrhagic telangiectasia)

CLINICAL SIGNS
- Multiple telangiectasia on the face, lips and buccal mucosa
- Anaemia: gastrointestinal bleeding
- Cyanosis and chest bruit: pulmonary vascular abnormality/shunt

DISCUSSION
- Autosomal dominant
- Increased risk of gastrointestinal haemorrhage, epistaxis and haemoptysis
- Vascular malformations:
  - Pulmonary shunts
  - Intracranial aneurysms: subarachnoid haemorrhage

Sickle cell disease

Examine this 25-year-old Afro-Caribbean female who has been admitted with chest and bone pain in association with worsening shortness of breath.

History

- **Sickle cell (vaso-occlusive) crisis:** sudden-onset bone pain and/or pleuritic chest pain – lasts days–weeks; acute chest syndrome: pneumonia-like illness
- **Anaemia:** long-standing fatigue with breathlessness on exertion, dizziness, syncope and headaches may worsen after infection
- **Complications:** infection (increased susceptibility due to functional hyposplenism, acute PE and pulmonary hypertension (ankle swelling), stroke/TIA (weakness, visual loss, seizures), leg ulcers, gall stones and priapism (males)
- **Triggers:** viral prodrome, cold weather, dehydration, alcohol and smoking, psychological stress/strenuous exercise, hypoxia, e.g. altitude (air travel), pregnancy
- **Family planning:** hydroxycarbamide is teratogenic, increased risk of crisis and miscarriage during pregnancy, genetic counselling

Examination

- Fever
- Dyspnoeic
- Jaundice
- Pale conjunctiva
- Raised JVP, parasternal heave, pansystolic murmur loudest at left sternal edge (tricuspid regurgitation) if pulmonary hypertension
- Reduced chest expansion due to pain with coarse expiratory crackles
- Small, crusted ulcers on lower third of legs

Discussion

- **Autosomal recessive** pattern of inheritance – heterozygote HbAS carriers (trait – asymptomatic); homozygote HbSS (disease)
- Vaso-occlusive crisis occurs as a result of sickling in the small vessels of any organ; lungs, kidney and bone most common
- Often precipitated by a viral illness, exercise or hypoxia
- Leg ulcers are due to ischaemia
- High mortality associated with the development of chest crises in adulthood
- Worse prognosis for patients with triad of leg ulcers, priapism and pulmonary hypertension

INVESTIGATIONS

- Blood tests: low Hb; high WCC and CRP; renal impairment; sickling on blood film
- CXR: linear atelectasis in a chest crisis; cardiomegaly: cardiac size proportional to degree of longstanding anaemia
- Urinalysis: microscopic haematuria if renal involvement in crisis
- Arterial blood gas: type I respiratory failure
- ECG and echo: dilated right ventricle with impaired systolic function; raised peak tricuspid regurgitant velocity
- CTPA: linear atelectasis with patchy consolidation ± acute pulmonary embolism

TREATMENT OF CRISIS

- Oxygen ± continuous positive airways pressure
- IV fluids
- Analgesia
- Antibiotics if evidence of infection

- Blood transfusion/exchange transfusion depending on degree of anaemia and severity of crisis
- May need further investigation of possible pulmonary hypertension if raised peak tricuspid regurgitant velocity, including right heart catheterization, after the acute event

PREVENTION/ADVICE
- Drink plenty of fluids
- Warm clothes, avoid sudden temperature changes
- NSAIDs and paracetamol
- Hydroxycarbamide or exchange transfusion programme if frequent crises or other features suggestive of a poor prognosis
- Long-term treatment with folic acid (increased haematopoiesis)
- Penicillin prophylaxis and vaccinations in patients with functional hyposplenism
- Educate when to seek medical attention, e.g. severe pain or breathlessness, D&V, weakness, seizure

PROGNOSIS
- HbSS survival ≈40–50 years old
- Worse prognosis with frequent chest crises or following development of pulmonary hypertension

Glandular fever

A 20-year-old man presents to A&E with a three-week history of fever, lethargy and cervical lymphadenopathy. He is referred to the Medical team for review.

- **Diagnosis:** EBV (glandular fever)
- **Differential diagnoses:** Other viral infections, lymphoma

History
- **Sore throat**
- Fevers
- Malaise and fatigue
- **Cervical lymphadenopathy**
- **Also ask about:**
  - 'Red flags' for
    - Complications of EBV – headaches (meningoencephalitis), ascending weakness (Guillain–Barré), jaundice (hepatitis)
    - Alternative diagnoses (lymphoma) – painless lymphadenopathy in multiple sites, night sweats, weight loss, alcohol-induced pain in lymph nodes
  - Travel, sexual and employment history
  - **Social contacts** with glandular fever: 'kissing disease'
  - Other medical issues, medication

Examination
- Jaundice
- Pallor and bruising (anaemia, thrombocytopenia complicating EBV)
- Throat – erythematous, palatal petechiae
- Cervical lymphadenopathy (and axillae, groin)
- Hepatosplenomegaly

Differential diagnosis
- Acute EBV infection with infectious mononucleosis (glandular fever)
- Hodgkin's lymphoma
- CMV
- HIV
- Viral hepatitis
- Toxoplasmosis

Discussion
INVESTIGATIONS
- **FBC and blood film** – lymphocytosis (atypical lymphocytes on film); also exclude anaemia, thrombocytopenia
- Test for **heterophile antibodies** (patient's serum agglutinates red blood cells from a different species – e.g. horse in the Monospot test); positive in about 90% of patients with EBV
- No further investigation needed if there is a clear clinical picture and positive heterophile antibody test
- Other investigations to consider if the diagnosis is unclear or heterophile antibodies negative:
  - EBV-specific antibodies
  - EBV PCR

- CMV PCR, HIV Ag/Ab, hepatitis serology
- Lymphoma work-up: tissue diagnosis: lymph-node biopsy/bone marrow; staging (lymph-node distribution in relation to diaphragm/organ/bone-marrow involvement): CXR, CT, MRI, PET

TREATMENT
- Symptomatic treatment: paracetamol, oral fluids
- Avoid contact sports for four weeks (risk of splenic rupture)
- Avoid amoxicillin – causes a generalized maculopapular rash in those with acute EBV

Nephrotic syndrome

This 58-year-old male complains of increasing bilateral leg swelling over the previous two months. His serum albumin is low at 18 g/L but all other baseline blood tests are normal. I have started him on frusemide 40 mg od. Thank you for assessing him.

History
- Duration and extent of oedema
- Associated symptoms – frothy urine
- Other co-morbidity – e.g. diabetes (diabetic nephropathy), SLE, rheumatoid arthritis, medications (see What Are the Common Causes?)
- Complications – especially venous thromboembolism (precipitated by the underlying diagnosis)

Differential diagnosis for bilateral leg oedema
- Cardiac failure
- Liver failure (hypoalbuminaemia)
- Nephrotic syndrome (hypoalbuminaemia)
- Fluid overload (e.g. advanced CKD)
- Inferior vena cava compression (intra-abdominal malignancy)

Examination
- Confirm the extent of the oedema
- Look for other signs of volume status – JVP, (postural) BP; patients with nephrotic syndrome are often underfilled
- Look for complications – DVT, bacterial skin infection, pleural effusions
- Look for an underlying cause, e.g. joint deformities in rheumatoid arthritis
- **You must state that you want to perform urinalysis!**

Discussion
INVESTIGATIONS
- **Urinalysis** and quantify proteinuria – either by urine albumin : creatinine ratio (uACR) or protein : creatinine ratio (uPCR); 24 h collections for proteinuria are now rarely used
- **Renal function**
- LFTs and BFTs
- FBC and coagulation
- Lipids
- Investigations for the underlying cause:
  - Autoimmune serology – ANA, complement, consider anti-phospholipase A2 receptor (PLA2R) antibodies in membranous nephropathy)
  - Infections – HIV, HBV, HCV
  - HbA1c
- CXR – fluid overload, malignancy
- Renal tract ultrasound
- **Renal biopsy** remains the gold standard
- Investigation for an underlying malignancy may be indicated

MANAGEMENT
- **Loop diuretics** (frusemide/bumetanide) – combined with fluid and salt restriction, daily weights to assess progress
- **Anticoagulation** – consider if serum albumin <20 g/L, as this is when thrombotic risk is highest
- Treat primary cause – guided by biopsy results
- ACE inhibitors and ARB reduce proteinuria
- SGLT2 inhibitors in selected cases (e.g. IgA nephropathy)

- Hypoalbuminaemia + proteinuria (>3 g/day or uACR >250 mg/mmol) + oedema
- Often associated with:
  - Hypercholesterolaemia
  - Increased thrombotic risk
  - Increased susceptibility to encapsulated bacterial infections

- **Primary glomerulonephritis**
  - Adults – membranous nephropathy, focal segmental glomerulosclerosis (FSGS), minimal change disease, IgA nephropathy
  - Children and young adults – minimal change disease
- **Secondary glomerular lesion** (due to a systemic disease):
  - Diabetic nephropathy
  - Amyloidosis
  - SLE
  - Rheumatoid arthritis
  - Drugs – NSAIDs, penicillamine, gold, heroin
  - Infections – HIV, HBV, HCV, malaria
  - Malignancy – solid organ tumours, leukaemia, lymphoma, myeloma

Jaundice

Please could you assess this 57-year-old man who has a background of primary sclerosing cholangitis. He has become jaundiced. His blood tests show an elevated ALP and bilirubin.

History
- Known liver disease (PSC)
  - When diagnosed?
  - When did he last have any blood tests and imaging (usually MRCP)?
  - Previous and current therapy (e.g. immunosuppression)
  - Associated conditions (50% will have **inflammatory bowel disease**, usually ulcerative colitis)
- Recent symptoms:
  - Jaundice
  - Weight loss
  - Abdominal pain
  - Abdominal swelling (ascites)
  - Fever
  - Anorexia
  - Pruritis
  - Drowsiness, daytime somnolence, cognitive problems (encephalopathy)
  - Change in bowel habit: melaena – tarry motions
  - Dark urine
- Risk factors for other new liver pathology:
  - New medications (e.g. antibiotics, herbal remedies and drug-induced liver injury)
  - **Alcohol use**
  - Viral infections (hepatitis)
    - Hepatitis A and E – faeco-oral, shellfish
    - Hepatitis B and C – IVDU, sexual, blood products
  - Travel and sexual history – risk of viral hepatitis; loss of libido
  - Tattoos and acupuncture
- Remember to take a **full medication history**

Examination
- General inspection – jaundice, stigmata of cirrhotic liver disease, e.g. spider naevi
- Cachexia
- Scratch marks, tattoos, IVDU
- Lymphadenopathy
- Abdominal examination: **hepatomegaly** – may be tender; **ascites** – shifting dullness, other masses
- Oedema
- Portal hypertension: caput medusae, haemorrhoids (no need to check in the exam!)
- Encephalopathy – GCS, orientation time/place/person, liver flap

Differential diagnosis
- Progression of PSC to cirrhosis
- Development of a new biliary stricture
- Cholelithiasis (1/3 of PSC patients develop gallstones)
- Cholangiocarcinoma (the most common malignancy developing in patients with PSC, with a 10–15% lifetime risk) – rapid onset of jaundice, weight loss and abdominal pain
- Hepatocellular carcinoma
- Gallbladder cancer
- Bowel cancer – increased risk if PSC + UC

Discussion

INVESTIGATIONS

- Repeat **liver function tests** with GGT, U&E, FBC (low Hb/platelets), calcium, **clotting**
- CXR (effusions, metastases)
- **Ultrasonography of liver** and biliary tree – dilated ducts, gallstones, mass lesions
- Depending on clinical context:
  - Hepatitis serology
  - Paracetamol levels
  - **MRCP and/or ERCP** (e.g. if suspecting cholangiocarcinoma, strictures, gallstones) – may be both diagnostic and therapeutic
  - OGD for varices – diagnostic and therapeutic
  - CT abdomen
  - Ascitic tap: WCC, protein, culture
- If encephalopathic investigate for reversible causes, e.g. dehydration, infection, GI bleed, constipation

TREATMENT

- Supportive treatment while under investigation:
  - **Diet:** high protein/calorie, low salt, abstinence from alcohol
  - Consider treating for **EtOH withdrawal/thiamine** and/or **N-acetyl cysteine** depending on cause
  - **Consider vitamin K** to ensure replete – will not correct coagulopathy unless deficient
- Complications of CLD:
  - **Ascites:** low-salt diet**,** diuretics – spironolactone/furosemide; paracentesis with albumin plasma expander to avoid haemodynamic collapse
  - **Spontaneous bacterial peritonitis:** IV antibiotics, prophylactic afterwards
  - **Varices:** propranolol/banding; **if bleeding** – IV antibiotics, octreotide/terlipressin bridges to OGD
  - **Encephalopathic:** lactulose, stop sedatives, empirical IV antibiotics
- Patient education and support
- Early discussion with local gastroenterology or liver unit
- If cholangiocarcinoma, prognosis is poor, although liver transplantation may be curative (but few patients are suitable)

Inflammatory bowel disease

This 36-year-old male has had bloody diarrhoea intermittently for the past six weeks. He has lost about 3 kg in weight.

History
- Gastrointestinal symptoms
  - Duration
  - Precipitants (travel, antibiotics, infectious contacts, foods, sexual history)
  - Stool frequency and consistency (Bristol stool scale)
  - Blood: fresh PR/mixed with stools
  - Mucus/slime
  - Urgency, incontinence, tenesmus
  - Abdominal pain, bloating: and association with eating, defecation
- Systemic symptoms
  - Fever, anorexia, weight loss, pruritis (PSC), fatigue
  - Rash, arthralgia, aphthous ulcers
- Family history

Examination
- General
  - Pallor/anaemia
  - Nutritional status
  - Pulse and BP
  - Oral ulceration
- Abdomen
  - Surgical scars, including current/past stoma sites
  - Tenderness
  - Palpable masses (e.g. right iliac fossa mass in Crohn's disease or colonic tumour in UC)
  - Ask to examine for perianal disease
  - Signs of chronic liver disease: jaundice and hepatosplenomegaly (PSC) in UC
- Skin
  - See Erythema Nodosum
- Evidence of treatment
  - Steroid side effects
  - Ciclosporin (gum hypertrophy and hypertension)
  - Hickman lines/scars

Discussion
INVESTIGATION
- Stool microscopy and culture: exclude infective cause of diarrhoea
- FBC and inflammatory markers: monitor disease activity
- AXR: exclude toxic dilatation in UC and small bowel obstruction due to strictures in Crohn's
- Sigmoidoscopy/colonoscopy and biopsy: histological confirmation
- Bowel contrast studies: strictures and fistulae in Crohn's disease
- Further imaging: white cell scan and CT scan

Cause
- Genetic, environmental and other factors combine to produce an exaggerated, sustained and mucosal inflammatory response

Differential diagnosis
- Crohn's: *Yersinia*, tuberculosis, lymphoma (and UC)
- UC: infection (e.g. *Campylobacter* spp), ischaemia, drugs and radiation (and Crohn's)
- Irritable bowel syndrome (IBS): bloating, gas, but weight stable, no bloody diarrhoea

TREATMENT

	Crohn's	UC
Mild–moderate disease	Oral steroid	Oral or topical (rectal steroid)
	5-ASA	5-ASA (e.g. mesalazine)
Severe disease	IV steroid	IV steroid
	IV infliximab	IV ciclosporin
Maintenance therapy	Oral steroid	Oral steroid
	Azathioprine	5-ASA
	Methotrexate	Azathioprine
	TNFα inhibitors: infliximab, adalimumab	

- **Medical:**
  - Antibiotics (metronidazole): in Crohn's with perianal infection, fistulae or small bowel bacterial overgrowth
  - Nutritional support: high-fibre, elemental and low-residue diets
  - Psychological support
- **Surgical:**
  - Crohn's: obstruction from strictures, complications from fistulae and perianal disease and failure to respond to medical therapy
  - UC: chronic symptomatic relief, emergency surgery for severe refractory colitis and colonic dysplasia or carcinoma

Complications:

Crohn's disease	Ulcerative colitis
Malabsorption	Anaemia
Anaemia	Toxic dilatation
Abscess	Perforation
Fistula	Colonic carcinoma
Intestinal obstruction	

Colonic carcinoma and UC
- Higher risk in patients with pancolitis (5–10% at 15–20 years) and in those with PSC
- Surveillance: 3-yearly colonoscopy for patients with pancolitis >10 years, increasing in frequency with every decade from diagnosis (2-yearly 20–30 years, annually >30 years)
- Colectomy if dysplasia is detected

Primary sclerosing cholangitis and UC
- Diagnosis: LFTs, MRI, ERCP, liver biopsy
- Treatment: pruritis – bile sequestrants, antihistamines, opiates; bile duct angioplasty/ stent; liver transplant

Extra-intestinal manifestations:

Mouth	Aphthous ulcers*
Skin	Erythema nodosum* Pyoderma gangrenosum (UC)* Finger clubbing*
Joint	Large joint arthritis* Seronegative arthritides
Eye	Uveitis,* episcleritis* and iritis*
Liver	Primary sclerosing cholangitis (UC) Systemic amyloidosis

* Related to disease activity.

Infectious (traveller's) diarrhoea
This 26-year-old male has had diarrhoea since returning from Africa three weeks ago.

History
- Duration, severity: frequency and volume, fever, vomiting, tenesmus; **bloody/watery**
- Weight loss
- **Travel history:** particularly low socioeconomic countries – Africa, India, South America
- Contact history
- Drug history: antibiotics
- Ingestion unfiltered water, raw or undercooked food (food poisoning notify UKHSA)
- **Employment history:** daycare worker, food handler (notify UKHSA), health worker
- Medical history – IBS (main differential diagnosis), immunosuppression, prosthetic joint/valve, haemoglobinopathy (HbSS)

Examination
- Dehydration: skin turgor, dry mucous membranes, tachycardia, hypotension, focal or diffuse abdominal tenderness

Discussion
- Very common – second most common reason that travellers seek medical attention

Causes: triage into bloody and non-bloody diarrhoea (bold notify UKHSA)

	Non-bloody	Bloody
Bacteria	Enterotoxigenic *E. coli* (traveller's diarrhoea)	***Campylobacter* spp**
	***Salmonella* spp, *Shigella* spp, *Yersinia* spp**	*E. coli* producing Shiga-like toxin, e.g. *E. coli* O157:H7
Virus	Norovirus (commonest)	
	Rotavirus	
Parasite	***Giardia lambia***	***Entamoeba histolytica***
	Cryptosporidium	
Toxin	*Clostridium difficile, Staphylococcus aureus*	

MANAGEMENT
- **Usually self-limiting** – oral/intravenous hydration/electrolytes; loperamide
- FBC, U&E, Cr, CRP; blood culture; **stool testing:** >1 day, bloody stool with fever, dehydration, signs of sepsis, recent antibiotic use or important to public health (food handler); if travel also look for ova and parasites
- Pathogen-directed treatment:
  - Unjustified for mild disease, risk of antibiotic resistance (except immunosuppressed) and commonly viral

- ○ Non-traveller non-bloody diarrhoea with antibiotic use: metronidazole; fever/moderate–severe: ciprofloxacin
- ○ Traveller non-bloody diarrhoea (particularly SE Asia): azithromycin
- ○ Bloody diarrhoea: fever/moderate–severe: ciprofloxacin
- *E. coli* O157 and haemolytic uraemic syndrome: blood film: schistocytes (red cell fragments), low platelets; supportive treatment: steroid, dialysis, blood transfusion
- Registered medical practitioners have a **statutory duty to notify the UKHSA** of certain infectious diseases

Swollen calf

This 34-year-old female patient has a swollen right leg. Her only medication is the OCP.

- **Diagnosis:** deep vein thrombosis
- **Differential diagnosis:** ruptured Baker's cyst, cellulitis, muscular strain, chronic venous insufficiency

History

SYMPTOMS OF DVT
- Unilateral swollen, red and tender calf

RISK FACTORS OF DVT
- Medical conditions, e.g. active cancer or heart failure (prothrombotic states)
- Immobility, e.g. flight, surgery (especially orthopaedic), stroke, etc.
- Previous personal or family history of DVT or PE
- Pregnancy
- Oral contraceptive use in women
- Inflammatory bowel disease and nephrotic syndrome

DIFFERENTIAL DIAGNOSIS
- Previous knee trauma or joint problem

COMPLICATIONS
- PE: pleuritic chest pain or breathlessness consistent with PE

TREATMENT CONSIDERATIONS
- Bleeding: contraindication to oral anticoagulation

Examination

CONFIRM THE DIAGNOSIS OF DVT
- Calf swelling (10 cm below the tibial tuberosity) >3 cm difference
- Deep calf tenderness
- Superficial venous engorgement and pitting oedema
- Tenderness along deep veins, e.g. in thigh

ELICIT A CAUSE
- Examine abdomen and pelvis (exclude mass compressing veins)

SIGNS OF COMPLICATIONS
- Thrombophlebitis: local tenderness and erythema
- Pulmonary embolus: pleural rub and right heart failure

TREATMENT CONSIDERATIONS
Peripheral pulses for compression stockings

Discussion

INVESTIGATIONS
- Calculate the pre-test probability – e.g. Wells' score
- **D-dimer** (sensitive but not specific test – can rule out diagnosis if negative in low/ intermediate pre-test probability)
- **Compression ultrasound**

- Urinalysis
- Pregnancy test
- FBC, INR
- Consider seeking underlying cause if suspected:
  - CXR (malignancy/also if suspect PE)
  - Thrombophilia screen if recurrent or positive family history
  - CT abdomen/pelvis if aged >50 years, recent weight loss, or other symptoms/signs
  - Mammography in females
  - PR and PSA in men

TREATMENT
- **Anticoagulation:**
  - Duration: 3 months first DVT, lifelong if recurrent
  - Anticoagulant choice: DOAC (apixaban, rivaroxaban are first-line), also warfarin, low molecular weight heparin
- Provide patient information leaflet and advice about anticoagulation
- Compression stockings may reduce post-phlebitic syndrome

Leg ulcers

Please review this 72-year-old male patient who has leg ulcers. He has been treated in the community for some time but I am now concerned that they have become infected and he has not responded to oral antibiotics.

- **Diagnosis:** venous leg ulcer
- **Differential:** arterial or diabetic (neuropathic) leg ulcer

History
DESCRIBE SYMPTOMS
- Pain: arterial (venous and neuropathic are painless)
- Location

ASSOCIATED DISEASES
- Venous: DVT, chronic venous insufficiency, varicose veins, CCF
- Arterial: PVD
- Neuropathic: sensory neuropathy, diabetes

COMPLICATIONS
- Infection:
  - Localised – ulcer; and surrounding skin – cellulitis
  - Spreading – tracking along lymphatic drainage with lymphadenopathy
  - Systemic – bacteraemia/septicaemia

Examination
VENOUS
- Gaiter area of lower leg
- **Stigmata of venous hypertension:** varicose veins or scars from vein stripping, oedema, lipodermatosclerosis, varicose eczema, atrophie blanche
- Pelvic/abdominal mass
- Think of intravenous drug abuse if groin cellulitis/sinus at injection site
- Lymphadenopathy if chronic infection

ARTERIAL
- Distal extremities and pressure points
- Trophic changes: hairless and paper-thin shiny skin
- Cold with poor capillary refill
- **Peripheral pulses absent**

NEUROPATHIC
- Pressure areas, e.g. under the metatarsal heads
- **Peripheral neuropathy** – determine sensory level
- Charcot's joints

COMPLICATIONS
- **Infection:** temperature, pus and cellulitis, tracking
- **Malignant change:** Marjolin's ulcer (squamous cell carcinoma)

Discussion
OTHER CAUSES OF A LEG ULCER
- Vasculitic, e.g. rheumatoid arthritis
- Neoplastic, e.g. squamous cell carcinoma
- Infectious, e.g. syphilis
- Haematological, e.g. sickle cell anaemia
- Tropical, e.g. cutaneous leishmaniasis

INVESTIGATIONS
- Doppler ultrasound
- Ankle–brachial pressure index (0.8–1.2 is normal, <0.8 implies arterial insufficiency)
- Arteriography

TREATMENT
- Specialist nurse: wound care
- **Venous:**
  - Four-layer compression bandaging (if no PVD)
  - Varicose vein surgery
- **Arterial:**
  - Angioplasty or vascular reconstruction/amputation

CAUSES OF NEUROPATHIC ULCERS
- Diabetes mellitus
- Tabes dorsalis
- Syringomyelia

Red rashes

This patient has a red rash – please assess.

These cases are often spot diagnoses.

DIAGNOSIS: PSORIASIS

History

DESCRIBE THE RASH
- Location, appearance, pruritis

PSYCHOSOCIAL IMPACT
- Particularly important in young women
- Confidence, relationships, work
- Depression

EXACERBATING FACTORS
- Stress, alcohol, cigarettes, drugs (β-blockers), trauma

TREATMENT
- PUVA: risk of melanoma (fair skin, family history)
- Immunosuppression: intercurrent infections
- Systemic side effects: steroids
- If pregnant: some treatments are teratogenic

Examination

RASH
- Chronic plaque (classical) type: multiple, well-demarcated, **'salmon-pink'**, scaly plaques on **extensor** surface
- Check behind ears, scalp and umbilicus
- Koebner phenomenon: plaques at sites of trauma
- Skin staining from treatment

NAILS
- Pitting, onycholysis, hyperkeratosis, discoloration

JOINTS
- **Psoriatic arthropathy** (10%), five forms:
  - DIPJ involvement (similar to OA)
  - Large joint mono-/oligoarthritis
  - Seronegative (similar to RA)
  - Sacroiliitis (similar to ankylosing spondylitis)
  - Arthritis mutilans

Discussion

DEFINITION
- Epidermal hyperproliferation and accumulation of inflammatory cells

TREATMENT
- **Topical** (in- or outpatient):
  - **Emollients**
  - **Calcipotriol**
  - **Coal tar**
  - Stains brown

- ○ **Dithranol**
  - ○ Stains purple and burns normal skin
- ○ **Hydrocortisone**
- **Phototherapy:**
  - ○ UVB
  - ○ Psoralen + UVA (PUVA)
- **Systemic:**
  - ○ **Cytotoxics** (methotrexate and ciclosporin)
  - ○ **Anti-TNFα** (adalimumab, etanercept, infliximab)
  - ○ **Retinoids** (acitretin): teratogenic

COMPLICATIONS
- **Erythroderma:** life-threatening
- **Systemic side-effects of steroid/cytotoxics**

CAUSES OF NAIL PITTING
- **Psoriasis**
- Lichen planus
- Alopecia areata
- Fungal infections

KOEBNER PHENOMENON SEEN WITH
- **Psoriasis**
- Lichen planus
- Viral warts
- Vitiligo
- Sarcoid

DIAGNOSIS: ECZEMA

History
DESCRIBE THE RASH
- Location, appearance, pruritis

PSYCHOSOCIAL IMPACT
- Particularly important in young women
- Confidence, relationships, work
- Depression

ATOPIC (ENDOGENOUS)
- Asthma, hay fever and allergy

ENVIRONMENTAL (EXOGENOUS)
- Primary irritant dermatitis: may just affect hands
- What is their job?

Examination
RASH
- **Erythematous and lichenified** patches of skin
- Predominantly **flexor** aspects of joints
- Fissures (painful), especially hands and feet
- Excoriations
- Secondary bacterial infection

- Respiratory: polyphonic wheeze (asthma)

SYSTEMIC TREATMENT EFFECTS
- Steroids: e.g. blood pressure, diabetes, osteoporosis

Discussion
INVESTIGATIONS
- Patch testing for allergies

TREATMENT
- Avoid precipitants
- **Topical:**
  - Emollients
  - Steroids
  - Tacrolimus: small increased risk of Bowen's disease
- Antihistamines for pruritis
- Antibiotics for secondary infection
- **UV light therapy**
- Systemic immunosuppression therapy in severe cases: prednisolone, methotrexate, ciclosporin, MMF, IL-4 antagonists, e.g. dupilumab

DIAGNOSIS: ERYTHEMA NODOSUM

History
SKIN
- Tender, red, smooth, shiny nodules on the shins

SCREEN FOR CAUSE
- Sarcoidosis
- Streptococcal throat infection
- Streptomycin, sulphonamides
- Oral contraceptive pill
- Pregnancy
- TB
- Inflammatory bowel disease
- Lymphoma
- Idiopathic

Examination
RASH
- **Tender, red, smooth, shiny nodules** commonly found on the **shins** (although anywhere with subcutaneous fat)
- Older lesions leave a bruise

JOINTS
- Tenderness and swelling

CAUSE
- Red, sore throat (streptococcal infection)
- Parotid swelling (sarcoidosis)

Discussion
- Pathology: granulomatous inflammation of subcutaneous fat (panniculitis)
- Other skin manifestations of sarcoidosis:
  - ○ **Nodules and papules:** red/brown seen particularly around the face, nose, ears and neck; demonstrates Koebner's phenomenon
  - ○ **Lupus pernio:** diffuse bluish/brown plaque with central small papules commonly affecting the tip of the nose

DIAGNOSIS: HENOCH–SCHÖNLEIN PURPURA

History
TRIAD
- **Purpuric rash**: usually on **extensor** surfaces of buttocks and legs
- **Arthralgia**
- **Abdominal pain**

PRECIPITANTS
- Infections: streptococci, HSV, parvovirus B19, etc.
- Drugs: antibiotics

COMPLICATIONS
- Renal involvement (IgA nephropathy): visible or non-visible haematuria, proteinuria
- Hypertension

Examination
RASH
- Purpuric rash: usually on buttocks and legs

JOINTS
- Inflammation in the hand joints

OTHER
- Blood pressure
- Urine dipstick – blood and protein
- Ask to check renal function

Discussion
- Small-vessel vasculitis: IgA and C3 deposition
- Normal or raised platelet count (distinguishes from other forms of purpura)
- Children > adults, males > females

TREATMENT
- Most **spontaneously recover** without treatment, although steroids may help recovery and treat painful arthralgia

PROGNOSIS
- 90% full recovery although can recur

Skin malignancy
This Caucasian patient has noticed a lump on their face and is concerned about its appearance.

- **Diagnosis:** basal cell carcinoma
- **Differential:** malignant melanoma, squamous cell carcinoma, actinic keratosis

History
SYMPTOMS
- Location and rapidity of growth
- Recent changes or bleeding

RISK FACTORS
- Sun exposure
- Occupation: exposure to dust/chemicals, outdoor work
- Family or past medical history of skin cancer

ASSOCIATIONS
- Solid organ transplant: immunosuppression

COMPLICATIONS
- Local invasion or metastasis: bone pain, neurological or abdominal problems

Basal cell carcinoma
- Usually on face/trunk: sun-exposed areas
- **Pearly nodule with rolled edge**
- Superficial telangiectasia
- Ulceration in advanced lesions
- Other lesions

NATURAL HISTORY
- **Slowly grow** over a few months
- **Local invasion only**, rarely metastasize

TREATMENT
- Curettage/cryotherapy if superficial
- Surgical excision ± radiotherapy

Squamous cell carcinoma
- Sun-exposed areas (+ lips + mouth)
- Actinic keratoses: pre-malignant (red and scaly patches)
- Varied appearance
  - Keratotic nodule
  - Polypoid mass
  - Cutaneous ulcer
- Other lesions/previous scars
- Metastases (draining lymph nodes/hepatomegaly/bone tenderness)

Squamous cell carcinoma in situ (Bowen's disease)
DIAGNOSIS
- Biopsy suspicious lesions

TREATMENT
- Surgery ± radiotherapy
- 5% metastasize

Malignant melanoma

- Patient's appearance: mention risks
  - Fair skin with freckles
  - Light hair
  - Blue eyes
- **Appearance of lesion**
  - **A**symmetrical
  - **B**order irregularity
  - **C**olour (black: often irregular pigmentation, may be colourless)
  - **D**iameter >6 mm
  - **E**nlarging
- Other lesions/previous scars
- Metastases (draining lymph nodes/hepatomegaly/bone tenderness)

DIAGNOSIS/TREATMENT
- Excision
- Staged on Breslow thickness (maximal depth of tumour invasion into dermis):
  - <1.5 mm = 90% 5-year survival
  - >3.5 mm = 40% 5-year survival
- Sampling of draining lymph nodes
- Surveillance for low-risk node-negative disease
- High-risk and/or node-positive disease – immunotherapy with immune checkpoint inhibitors
- Beware the man with a glass eye and ascites: ocular melanoma!

Skin and hyperextensible joints

I'd like to refer this 54-year-old female patient with a skin problem and hypermobility.

- **Diagnosis: Pseudoxanthoma elasticum**

History
- Explore skin problems
  - Hereditary: chronic
- Other problems
  - Hyperextensible joints
  - Reduced visual acuity
  - Hypertension
  - MI or CVA
  - Gastric bleed
- Family history

Examination
SKIN
- **'Plucked chicken skin'** appearance: loose skin folds especially at the neck and axillae, with yellow pseudo-xanthomatous plaques

EYES
- Blue sclerae
- Retinal angioid streaks (cracks in Bruch's membrane) and macular degeneration

CARDIOVASCULAR
- Blood pressure: 50% are hypertensive
- Mitral valve prolapse: EC and PSM

Discussion
- Inheritance: 80% autosomal recessive (*ABCC6* gene, chromosome 16)
- Degenerative elastic fibres in skin, blood vessels and eye
- Premature coronary artery disease

- **Differential diagnosis: Ehlers–Danlos**

History
- As above
- No premature coronary disease
- Family history more apparent (autosomal dominant)

Examination
SKIN AND JOINTS
- Fragile skin: multiple ecchymoses, scarring – **'fish-mouth' scars** especially on the knees
- **Hyperextensible skin:** able to tent up skin when pulled (avoid doing this)
- Joint **hypermobility** and dislocation (scar from joint repair/replacement)

CARDIOVASCULAR
- Mitral valve prolapse
- Aortic dilatation – risk of dissection/rupture

ABDOMINAL
- Scars:
  - Aneurysmal rupture and dissection
  - Bowel perforation and bleeding

Discussion
- Inheritance: autosomal dominant
- Defect in collagen causing increased skin elasticity
- No premature coronary artery disease

Rheumatoid arthritis

This 35-year-old female has had painful, stiff fingers for some months. These are progressively get-ting worse and she has noticed some swelling of her hand joints. Her CRP is elevated at 35 mg/L and ESR 47 mm/h.

History
SYMPTOMS
- Joints involved, pain, function
- Early morning stiffness and pain – indicative of an inflammatory arthritis
- Functional impairment
- Other system involvement (see below)

DISABILITY AND HANDICAP
- Occupation and ADLs
- Sports and hobbies

DRUGS
- Will help assess disease activity – analgesics and DMARDs

SYSTEMIC EFFECTS OF DISEASE AND TREATMENT
- See below

Examination
OBSERVE HANDS (SLEEVES ROLLED BEYOND ELBOW)
- **Symmetrical and deforming polyarthropathy**
- Volar subluxation and ulnar deviation at the MCPJs
- Subluxation at the wrist
- Swan-neck deformity (hyperextension of the PIPJ and flexion of the DIPJ)
- Boutonnière's deformity (flexion of the PIPJ and hyperextension of the DIPJ)
- 'Z' thumbs
- Muscle wasting (disuse atrophy)
- Surgical scars:
  - Carpal tunnel release (wrist)
  - Joint replacement (especially thumb)
  - Tendon transfer (dorsum of hand)
- Rheumatoid nodules (elbows)

ASSESS DISEASE ACTIVITY
- **Active disease:** joint inflammation and synovitis – especially MCPJs and wrists
  - Look for inflamed joints, erythema
  - Feel for heat
  - The 'squeeze test' – gently compress across the MCPJs between your thumb and fingers; pain implies synovitis (although avoid this in the exam!)
  - Gently palpate each joint in turn from wrist down to DIPJs, feeling for synovitis and assessing for pain
- **Burnt-out disease:** often with the classical signs above (e.g. swan-neck deformity) but no signs of inflammation

ASSESS FUNCTION
- **Power grip:** 'squeeze my fingers'
- **Precision grip:** 'pick up a coin' or 'do up your buttons'
- **Key grip:** 'pretend to use this key'
- Remember the wheelchair, walking aids and splints

- Steroids: Cushingoid
- C-spine stabilization scars

- **Pulmonary:**
  - Pleural effusions
  - Fibrosing alveolitis
  - Obliterative bronchiolitis
  - Caplan's nodules
- **Eyes:**
  - Dry (secondary Sjögren's)
  - Scleritis
- **Neurological:**
  - Carpal tunnel syndrome (commonest)
  - Peripheral neuropathy
  - Atlanto-axial subluxation: quadriplegia
- **Haematological:**
  - Felty's syndrome: RA + splenomegaly + neutropenia
  - Anaemia (all types!)
- **Cardiac:**
  - Pericarditis
  - Coronary artery disease
- **Renal:**
  - Nephrotic syndrome (secondary amyloidosis or membraneous glomerulonephritis, e.g. due to penicillamine)

Main differential diagnosis
- Psoriatic arthropathy:
  - Nail changes
  - Psoriasis: elbows, behind ears and scalp

Discussion
- Elevated inflammatory markers (CRP and ESR)
- FBC (anaemia), renal function, urinalysis, serum albumin (if oedema)
- Serological tests
  - **Positive rheumatoid factor** (IgM against self-IgG) in 80% – also present in other inflammatory conditions and with increasing age (but no disease association)
  - **Anti-CCP** (cyclic citrullinated peptide) positive in about 80% of patients, but high specificity
- Radiological changes in affected joints:
  - Soft tissue swelling
  - Loss of joint space
  - Articular erosions
  - Periarticular osteoporosis
- CXR, CT thorax and lung function if respiratory involvement suspected

- Is clinical, but may use the American College of Rheumatology criteria that base diagnosis on a combination of:
  - Number of joints involved
  - Elevated inflammatory markers
  - Positive serological tests (rheumatoid factor or anti-CCP)
  - Prolonged duration of symptoms (>6 weeks)

TREATMENT
- **Medical**
  - Early introduction of **disease-modifying anti-rheumatoid drugs** (DMARDs) to suppress disease activity:
    - Methotrexate
    - Leflunamide
    - Sulphasalazine
    - Consider hydroxychloroquine for mild disease
    - These can be combined to achieve control
  - Steroids may be used in the short term to help manage pain and suppress flares of disease activity, but avoid long-term use
  - NSAIDs may also be used for pain/stiffness
  - Ongoing disease activity (having failed DMARDs alone or in combination) may require **immunomodulation therapy:**
    - **Anti-TNF therapy:** infliximab/etanercept/adalimumab; screen for TB and hepatitis B before use; side effects include rash, opportunistic infections
    - **B cell depletion therapy:** rituximab (anti-CD20 mAb)
    - **Anti IL-6:** rocilizumab
- **Supportive**
  - Explanation and education
  - Exercise and physiotherapy
  - Occupational therapy and social support
- **Surgery**
  - Joint replacement, tendon transfer, etc.

PROGNOSIS
- 5 years – 1/3 unable to work; 10 years – 1/2 significant disability

Side effects and monitoring of RA treatment:

	Serious side effects	Monitor
Methotrexate	Neutropenia, pulmonary toxicity and hepatitis	CXR, FBC, LFT
Hydroxychloroquine	Retinopathy	Visual acuity
Sulphasalazine	Rash and bone marrow suppression	FBC
Corticosteroids	Osteoporosis	
Azathioprine	Neutropenia	FBC
Gold complexes	Thrombocytopenia, rash	FBC
Penicillamine	Proteinuria, thrombocytopenia rash	FBC and urine

Systemic lupus erythematosus

Please see this 49-year-old female with a red rash on her face. She also complains of dry eyes.

History

DESCRIBE THE RASH
- Location, appearance, other areas affected
- **Photosensitivity**
- Flares and remission or permanent
- If isolated without other conditions consider rosacea (particularly if fair-skinned)

ASSOCIATED CONDITIONS
- Constitutional symptoms including fever, weight loss, fatigue
- Cold hands: **Raynaud's phenomenon**
- Dry eyes/mucous membranes: **Sjögren's syndrome**
- PMH – DVT, PE, stroke and MI: **anti-phospholipid syndrome** (APS)
- Pale, fatigue, breathlessness: anaemia of chronic disease
- Fatigue, weight gain, cold sensitivity: hypothyroidism (also sometimes hyperthyroidism)

PSYCHOSOCIAL IMPACT
- Particularly important in young women
- Depression; reduced confidence: relationships, work
- Family planning: infertility/treatment teratogenicity; miscarriage (particularly with APS)

SYSTEMIC EFFECTS OF SLE OR TREATMENT
- Hypertension, joint pains, breathlessness, abdominal pain
- Immunosuppression: skin changes: blue/grey, psoriasiform/cancer/infections/Cushingoid

Examination

FACE
- **Malar 'butterfly' rash** – erythematous, flat or raised rash on cheeks and bridge of nose
- **Discoid rash** ± scarring (discoid lupus)
- **Oral ulceration** (painless)
- Scarring alopecia

HANDS
- Vasculitic lesions (nail-fold infarcts)
- Jaccoud's arthropathy – stiffness and pain (mimics RA but due to tendon contractures not joint destruction)

SYSTEMIC EFFECTS OF SLE
- Respiratory: percussion and auscultation
  - Pleural effusion with rub
  - Fibrosing alveolitis
- Cardiac:
  - Pericardial rub – pericarditis with effusion (commonest)
  - Valvular incompetence (Libman–Sacks endocarditis)
- Neurological: finger–nose–finger and/or pronator drift
  - Focal neurology
  - Chorea
  - Ataxia
- Renal:
  - Hypertension; urine dip

Discussion

- Serum autoantibodies (**ANA and anti-dsDNA** – highly sensitive)

DISEASE ACTIVITY
- Elevated ESR but normal CRP (raised CRP too indicates infection)
- Elevated immunoglobulins; reduced complement (C_4)
- U&Es, urine microscopy (glomerulonephritis)
- Consider: aPL antibody (APS), FBC, TFTs, 12-lead ECG, CXR, echo

DIAGNOSIS: 4/11 OF AMERICAN COLLEGE OF RHEUMATOLOGY CRITERIA
- Malar rash
- Discoid rash
- Photosensitivity
- Oral ulcers
- Arthritis
- Serositis (pleuritis or pericarditis)
- Renal involvement (proteinuria or cellular casts)
- Neurological disorder (seizures or psychosis)
- Haematological disorder (autoimmune haemolytic anaemia or pancytopenia)
- Immunological disorders (positive anti-dsDNA or anti-Sm antibodies)
- Elevated ANA titre

TREATMENT
- **Mild disease (cutaneous/joint involvement only):**
  - Topical corticosteroids
  - Hydroxychloroquine
- **Moderate disease (+ other organ involvement):**
  - Prednisolone
  - Azathioprine
- **Severe disease (+ severe inflammatory involvement of vital organs):**
  - Methylprednisolone
  - Mycophenolate mofetil (lupus nephritis)
  - Cyclophosphamide
  - Azathioprine
- With APS: consider aspirin (prophylaxis) or anticoagulation (after venous thrombosis)

CYCLOPHOSPHAMIDE SIDE EFFECTS
- **H**aematological and **h**aemorrhagic cystitis
- **I**nfertility
- **T**eratogenicity

PROGNOSIS
- Good: 90% survival at 10 years

Systemic sclerosis
This 54-year-old female has painful and swollen hands and also reports difficulty swallowing.

History
HANDS
- **Raynaud's phenomenon** (Raynaud's disease is idiopathic!); colour change order: white (vasoconstriction) → blue (cyanosis) → red (hyperaemia)
- Ask about function: how does the condition affect ADLs/work, etc.

FUNCTIONAL ENQUIRY
- Hypertension or heart problems
- Lung problems – cough, dyspnoea
- Swallowing problems or indigestion

Examination
HANDS
- Perfusion and any current evidence of Raynaud's
- **Sclerodactyly:** 'prayer sign'
- **Calcinosis** (may ulcerate)
- Assess function: holding a cup or pen

FACE
- **Tight skin**
- Beaked nose
- Microstomia
- **Peri-oral furrowing**
- **Telangiectasia**
- Alopecia

OTHER SKIN LESIONS
- Morphoea: focal/generalized patches of sclerotic skin
- En coup de sabre (scar down central forehead)

BLOOD PRESSURE
- **Hypertension**

RESPIRATORY
- **Interstitial fibrosis** (fine and bibasal crackles)

CARDIAC
- **Pulmonary hypertension** (RV heave, loud P_2 and TR)
- Evidence of failure
- Pericarditis (rub)

RENAL
- Urine dip: proteinuria

Discussion
CLASSIFICATION
- **Localized:** morphoea to patch of skin only
- **Systemic:** limited and **diffuse**

Limited systemic sclerosis	Diffuse systemic sclerosis
Distribution limited to below elbows and knees and face	Widespread cutaneous and early visceral involvement
Slow progression (years)	Rapid progression (months)
Many patients have features of the **CREST** syndrome: • **C**alcinosis • **R**aynaud's phenomenon • o**E**sophageal dysmotility • **S**clerodactyly • **T**elangiectasia	

INVESTIGATIONS
- **Autoantibodies:**
  - **ANA positive** (in 95%)
  - Anti-centromere antibody = limited disease (in 80%)
  - Scl-70 antibody = diffuse disease (in 70%)
  - Anti-RNA polymerase III antibody found in patients with diffuse disease, may indicate increased cancer risk
- **Hand radiographs:** calcinosis
- **Pulmonary disease: lower-lobe fibrosis and aspiration pneumonia:**
  - CXR, high-resolution CT scan and pulmonary function tests
- **Gastrointestinal disease: dysmotility and malabsorption**
  - FBC and B_{12}/folate
  - Endoscopy if severe reflux (not controlled with PPI)
  - Oesophageal manometry
  - Hydrogen breath test for bacterial overgrowth
- **Renal disease: glomerulonephritis**
  - U&E, urinalysis (mild proteinuria), haemolytic anaemia and consider renal biopsy
- **Cardiac disease: myocardial fibrosis and arrhythmias**
  - ECG and echo
  - Cardiac MRI
  - Right heart catheter – pulmonary hypertension

TREATMENT
- Symptomatic treatment only:
  - Camouflage creams
  - **Raynaud's therapy:**
    - Gloves, hand-warmers, etc.
    - Calcium-channel blockers
    - ACE inhibitors
    - Prostacyclin infusion (severe)
- **Renal:**
  - ACE inhibitors: treat/prevent hypertensive crisis, reduce mortality from renal failure
- **Gastrointestinal:**
  - Proton-pump inhibitor for oesophageal reflux

PROGNOSIS
- Diffuse systemic sclerosis: 50% survival to 5 years (most deaths are due to respiratory failure)

Ankylosing spondylitis
This 70-year-old male complains of back pain and reduced neck mobility.

History
- **Explore back symptoms**
  - **Back and joint pain/stiffness:** exacerbated by immobility and relieved with exercise, particularly at tendon insertion points (enthesitis) >3 months' duration
  - Reduced mobility
  - Flares, fever and fatigue

PSYCHOSOCIAL IMPACT
- Work, driving, ADLs, etc.

ASSOCIATED PROBLEMS
- Red, inflamed, painful eye: **anterior uveitis**
- Salmon pink rash, extensor surface with joint pain: **psoriasis** and **psoriatic arthropathy**
- Weight loss, bloody diarrhoea, abdominal pain: inflammatory bowel disease
- Weak legs, numbness genitals/anus, urinary retention: cauda equina syndrome (rare)
- Fragility fractures: osteoporosis
- Breathlessness: lung fibrosis, severe kyphosis – limiting chest expansion, heart failure (AR)
- Syncope: complete heart block

Examination
POSTURE
- **'?'** – fixed kyphoscoliosis, loss of lumbar lordosis and extension of cervical spine
- Protuberant abdomen, diaphragmatic breathing, reduced chest expansion (<5 cm girth)
- Increased occiput–wall distance (>5 cm)
- Reduced range of movement throughout entire spine
- **Schöber's test:** Two points marked 15 cm apart on the dorsal spine expand by less than 5 cm on maximum forward flexion

COMPLICATIONS
- **A**nterior uveitis (commonest 30%)
- **A**pical lung fibrosis
- **A**ortic regurgitation (4%): midline sternotomy
- **A**trio-ventricular nodal heart block (10%): pacemaker
- **A**rthritis (may be psoriatic arthropathy)

Discussion
GENETICS
- 90% association with **HLA B27**

INVESTIGATION
- Imaging: spine X-ray – vertebral fusion; MRI of sacroiliac joints – sacroiliitis

TREATMENT
- Exercise, physiotherapy and TENS
- Medical: analgesia, e.g. NSAIDs; disease modifiers: steroid, anti-TNF, mAb, JAK inhibitor
- Surgery: correct kyphosis, THR

Marfan's syndrome
Thank you for assessing this tall male patient with a murmur.

History
FAMILY HISTORY
- Functional enquiry:
  - Requirement for spectacles or eye surgery
  - Cardiac screening with echo or CT surveillance and surgery

Examination
GENERAL (SPOT DIAGNOSIS)
- **Tall** with **long extremities** (arm span > height)

HANDS
- **Arachnodactyly:** can encircle their wrist with thumb and little finger
- **Hyperextensible joints:** thumb able to touch ipsilateral wrist and adduct over the palm with its tip visible at the ulnar border

FACE
- **High-arched palate** with crowded teeth
- **Iridodonesis** (vibration of the iris with eye movement) is a marker of lens dislocation (ectopia lentis) – with **upward lens dislocation** visible on slit lamp examination

RESPIRATORY
- **Pectus** carinatum ('pigeon') or excavatum
- Scoliosis
- Scars from cardiac surgery or chest drains (pneumothorax)

CARDIAC
- Ascending dilatation and aortic valve incompetence: collapsing pulse
- Mitral valve prolapse
- Coarctation

ABDOMINAL
- Inguinal herniae and scars

CNS
- Normal cognition

Discussion
GENETICS
- Autosomal dominant and chromosome 15
- Defect in fibrillin protein (connective tissue)

MANAGEMENT
- **Surveillance:** monitoring of aortic root size with annual transthoracic echo
- **Treatment:**
  - β-blockers and angiotensin receptor blocker to slow aortic root dilatation (titrate to maximal tolerated dose)
  - pre-emptive aortic root surgery to prevent dissection and aortic rupture when diameter >5.0 cm or if growing rapidly (>1.0 cm/year)
- **Screen family members:** counselling and genetic screening of first-degree relatives, then echo

DIFFERENTIAL DIAGNOSIS
- Homocystinuria:
  - Marfanoid body habitus
  - Intellectual disability
  - Downward lens dislocation
  - Pro-thrombotic tendency

Paget's disease
This 75-year-old male patient has had numbness in his index finger and complains of deafness.

History
SYMPTOMS
- Usually asymptomatic change in bone shape
- Bone pain and tenderness (2%); headaches

ASSOCIATED CONDITIONS
- **Entrapment neuropathy:** carpal tunnel syndrome – median nerve distribution paraesthesia, visual problems, cauda equina syndrome, deafness
- Fragility fractures, associated osteoarthritis: joint pain and swelling
- CCF: breathlessness

Examination
- Bony enlargement: skull and long bones (**sabre tibia**)
- Deafness (conductive): **hearing aid**
- Pathological fractures: scars

CARDIAC
- High-output heart failure: elevated JVP, SOA, shortness of breath

NEURO
- Entrapment neuropathies: carpal tunnel syndrome – **positive Tinel's test:** tingling distal to median nerve tap
- **Fundi:** Optic atrophy and angioid streaks

Discussion
INVESTIGATIONS
- Grossly **elevated alkaline phosphatase**, normal calcium/phosphate
- Radiology:
  - 'Moth-eaten' on plain X-ray: **osteoporosis circumscripta**
  - **Increase uptake on bone scan**

TREATMENT
- Exercise, physiotherapy, occupational therapy (shoe inserts)
- Symptomatic: analgesia, hearing aid, carpal tunnel release, joint replacement
- Calcium/D$_3$, bisphosphonates

OTHER COMPLICATIONS
- Osteogenic sarcoma (1%)
- Basilar invagination (cord compression)
- Kidney stones

Causes of sabre tibia	Causes of angioid streaks
Paget's	Paget's
Osteomalacia	Pseudoxanthoma elasticum
Syphilis	Ehlers–Danlos

Other joint problems
This man has problems with painful hands (or knee or feet). Please assess him.

GOUT

History
CAUSE
- Diet and alcohol: **xanthine-rich foods** (meat/seafood/beer)
- Drugs: **diuretics**, calcineurin inhibitors (cyclosporin, tacrolimus)
- Other conditions: **chronic kidney disease**, **metabolic syndrome** (obesity, diabetes, hypertension)

Examination
- Asymmetrical swelling of the small joints of the hands and feet (commonly **first MTPJ**) – red/ purple, hot, tender
- Gouty tophi (chalky white deposits) seen around the joints, ear and tendons
- Reduced movement and function

ASSOCIATIONS
Obesity
- Hypertension
- Urate stones/nephropathy: nephrectomy scars
- Chronic renal failure: fistulae
- Solid organ transplant
- Lymphoproliferative disorders: lymphadenopathy

Discussion
CAUSE
- Urate excess

INVESTIGATION
- Uric acid levels (diagnostically unreliable at time of an acute flare)
- Synovial fluid: needle-shaped, negatively birefringent crystals
- Radiograph features: 'punched-out' periarticular changes

TREATMENT
- **Acute attack:**
  - Treat the cause, e.g. stop diuretic
  - Increase fluid intake
  - High-dose NSAIDs
  - Colchicine 0.5 mg bd
  - Steroid, e.g. oral prednisolone 30 mg od for 3–5 days
- **Prevention:**
  - Avoid precipitants
  - Allopurinol or febuxostat (xanthine oxidase inhibitors) – the goal is to titrate the dose to achieve suppression of serum urate (<300 µmol/L)
  - Losartan has a urate-lowering effect

OSTEOARTHRITIS

History
SYMPTOMS
- Morning stiffness (<30 min) ± weakness (disuse)
- Pain
- May be red or swollen during acute flare

- Assess function, ask about ADLs and work
- Mobility: walking stick, motorized wheelchair, etc.

PRIOR TREATMENTS
- Joint replacements
- NSAIDs: side effects – stomach ulcers, fluid retention, hypertension

DIFFERENTIAL DIAGNOSIS
- Traumatic fracture
- Rheumatoid arthritis: prolonged morning joint-related stiffness, systemic symptoms
- Septic arthritis: rapid-onset hot swollen joint, fever, systemic symptoms
- Bone malignancy: rapid-onset, persistent progressive pain especially at night
- Meniscal tear, cartilage problem: locking, 'giving way'
- Cruciate ligament: instability

Examination
- Asymmetrical distal interphalangeal joint deformity with **Heberden's nodes** (and sometimes **Bouchard's nodes** at the proximal interphalangeal joint)
- **Disuse atrophy** of hand muscles
- Crepitation, reduced movement and function
- Carpal tunnel syndrome or scars
- Other joint involvement and joint-replacement scars

Discussion
PREVALENCE
- 20% (common)

RADIOGRAPHIC FEATURES
- **Imaging is not needed** to make a diagnosis of OA
- X-ray: loss of joint space, osteophytes, peri-articular sclerosis and cysts
- CT or MRI may be helpful when planning surgery

TREATMENT
- **Weight reduction** if overweight
- **Exercise**, physiotherapy and occupational therapy (walking aids) – muscle strengthening
- Medical: **oral or topical NSAIDs**, interarticular steroid (short term)
- Surgical: **joint replacement** – deformity, loss of function, failed non-surgical management

Hypercalcaemia

Please assess this 76-year-old man who has been found to have a corrected calcium of 2.8 mmol/L on blood tests taken at the surgery.

History
- Symptoms of hypercalcaemia – **'bones, stones, abdominal groans and psychic moans':**
  - Sometimes none!
  - Mood disorder (fatigue, anxiety, depression)
  - Abdominal pain, constipation, nausea, vomiting, renal colic
  - Thirst, polyuria
  - Muscle weakness
- Symptoms relating to the underlying disease:
  - Malignancy – bone pain, cough, haemoptysis, weight loss
  - Sarcoidosis – dry cough
  - Addison's – other autoimmune conditions
- Past medical history and drug history

Examination
- 'Screening" exam if no clues from the history:
  - General inspection – cachexia, hydration status
  - Lymphadenopathy
  - Pleural effusion
  - Hepatomegaly, masses, ascites

Discussion
CAUSES
- **Primary hyperparathyroidism**
- **Malignancy:**
  - **Multiple myeloma**
  - Solid organ tumours with bony metastases
  - Solid organ tumours with production of PTH-related protein
- Medications:
  - Vitamin D and/or calcium supplements
  - Thiazide diuretics
  - Lithium
- Sarcoidosis
- Addison's disease
- Hyperthyroidism
- Prolonged immobility

INVESTIGATIONS
- Blood U&E, Cr, TFT, LFT, alkaline phosphatase, calcium (>2.6 mmol/L – corrected for serum albumin), phosphate, serum PTH, myeloma screen, serum ACE, random cortisol/ short Synacthen
- Urinary calcium
- CXR – masses, effusions, hilar lymphadenopathy
- If primary hyperparathyroidism confirmed: (para)thyroid ultrasound and Sesta-MIBI scan
- Consider CT imaging if suspected solid organ malignancy, renal imaging, bone mineral density imaging guided by presentation (do not investigate routinely)

TREATMENT
- Depends on level and other symptoms, but definitely if >3.0 mmol/L:
  - Intravenous rehydration
  - Intravenous bisphosphonates

Diabetes and complications

Diabetes may form the focus of a consultation or represent a significant co-morbidity. More detail is needed if it is the main theme.

General diabetes questions

- Type of diabetes: type I/II
- Duration
- Current and past treatment:
  - Injectable insulin (long- and short-acting, mixed)
  - Insulin pump
  - Oral hypoglycaemics (metformin, gliclazide, gliptins, SGLT2 inhibitors, etc.)
  - Other injectables (GLP-1 agonists)
  - Diet and weight loss
- Monitoring blood glucose and how: finger prick – capillary blood glucose, or a sensor (continuous glucose measurement – CGM)
- At what level of glucose do you experience symptoms of hypoglycaemia?
- How often do you have hypos – and when was the last time you needed someone else to help recognize and treat a hypo?
  - Triggers – diet, alcohol, treatment compliance, education, support
- Hospitalizations with diabetic issues (hypo- or hyperglycaemia, DKA)
- Complications of diabetes:
  - Medical (retinopathy, neuropathy, gastroparesis, etc.)
  - Psychosocial (work, relationships, body image)

Diabetes and the skin

This 48-year-old female has had type I diabetes mellitus for many years and now has a rash on her legs.

- **Diagnosis:** necrobiosis lipoidica diabeticorum
- **Differential:** diabetic dermopathy, granuloma annulare, leg ulcers, eruptive xanthomata, vitiligo, candidiasis

History

DIABETIC HISTORY/CARE
- Duration
- Insulin administration and glucose control: rotation of injection sites
- Foot care: podiatry

MICROVASCULAR COMPLICATIONS OF DIABETES
- Neuropathy
- Retinopathy

PSYCHOSOCIAL
- Impact on ability to work, form relationships, body image

Examination

SHINS
- **Necrobiosis lipoidica diabeticorum:**
  - Well-demarcated plaques with waxy-yellow centre and red–brown edges
  - Early: may resemble a bruise
  - Prominent skin blood vessels
  - Female preponderance (90%)
- **Diabetic dermopathy:**
  - Red/brown, atrophic lesions

FEET AND LEGS
- **Ulcers:** arterial or neuropathic (see Leg Ulcers)
- **Eruptive xanthomata:**
  - Yellow papules on buttocks and knees (also elbows)
  - Caused by hyperlipidaemia
- **Granuloma annulare:** flesh-coloured papules in annular configurations on the dorsum feet (and more commonly fingers) [/bl[

INJECTION SITES (THIGH)
- Lipoatrophy
- Fat hypertrophy

CUTANEOUS INFECTIONS
- Cellulitis
- Candidiasis (intertrigo): in skin creases

OTHER DISEASES
- Vitiligo (and other autoimmune diseases)
- Peripheral vascular disease: pulses
- Diabetic cheiroarthropathy – reduced hand function with joint stiffening and skin thickening, patients demonstrate the 'prayer sign' (unable to flatten hands together, like in prayer)

Discussion

TREATMENT FOR NECROBIOSIS LIPOIDICA DIABETICORUM
- Topical steroid and support bandaging
- Tight glycaemic control does not help

Xanthomata

- **Hypercholesterolaemia:** tendon xanthomata, xanthelasma and corneal arcus
- **Hypertriglyceridaemia:** eruptive xanthomata and lipaemia retinalis
- **Other causes of secondary hyperlipidaemia:**
  - Hypothyroidism
  - Nephrotic syndrome
  - Alcohol
  - Cholestasis

Diabetic retinopathy

This 66-year-old male patient with diabetes complains of blurred vision.

History
- Ask the patient to detail their problem: duration and nature of visual disturbance
- Establish any underlying medical diagnoses: especially presence or absence of diabetes
- Previous eye problems or treatment
- If they are diabetic: do they have regular (annual) retinal screening?

Examination
- Look around for clues: a white stick, braille book or glucometer
- **Fundoscopy:** check for red reflex (absent if mature cataract or vitreous haemorrhage)
  - Find the disc (infero-nasally) then follow each of the four main vessels out to the periphery of the quadrants, then ask the person to look up (examine superior retina), left and right (examining nasal and temporal retina depending on which eye) and down (examine inferior retina), and finish by examining the macular: 'look at the light'. It is much easier for the patient to look at a small spot size for viewing the macula if one is available on your ophthalmoscope
  - Check for **coexisting hypertensive changes** (they always ask!) – particularly AV nipping, which is more specific for hypertension

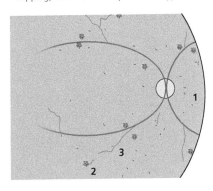

Background retinopathy ± maculopathy (R1M0 and R1M1)

1 Hard exudates
2 Flame and dot haemorrhages
3 Microaneurysms

Patients with background diabetic retinopathy are usually seen annually in the screening programme unless they also have signs of referable maculopathy (R1M1).

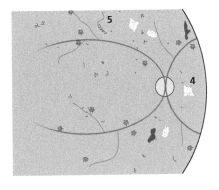

Pre-proliferative retinopathy ± maculopathy (R2M0 and R2M1).
Background changes plus:

4 Multiple cotton-wool spots – this is most dramatic but the least specific sign of pre-proliferative diabetic retinopathy and the NHS Diabetic Eye Screening Programme asks graders to look for the following three more specific signs of pre-proliferative diabetic retinopathy if multiple cotton-wool spots are present:
5 Multiple bot haemorrhages
6 Venous beading
7 Intraretinal microvascular abnormalities (IRMA)

Routine referral to ophthalmology.

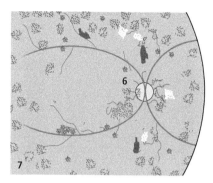

Proliferative retinopathy ± maculopathy (R3M0 and R3M1). Pre-proliferative changes plus:

8   Neovascularization of the disc (NVD) and/or
9   New vessels elsewhere (NVE)
10 Pan-retinal photocoagulation scars (from previous treatment)

Urgent referral to ophthalmology.

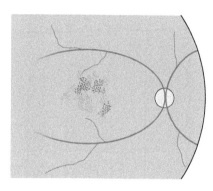

Diabetic maculopathy. Macular oedema or hard exudates within one disc space of the fovea. Routine referral to ophthalmology for most patients, with a small number with centre involvement and reduced vision (commonly blurring) requiring urgent referral to ophthalmology.

Discussion

SCREENING

- **Annual retinal screening** for all patients with diabetes (using retinal photography) with R and M level graded by the worst eye
- Refer to ophthalmology if pre-proliferative/proliferative diabetic retinopathy or clinically significant changes near the macula
- Background retinopathy usually occurs 10–20 years after diabetes is diagnosed
- The three highest risk factors for progression to sight-threatening diabetic retinopathy are the **current level of retinopathy** in the eye, the **duration of diabetes** and the **control of diabetes**

TREATMENT

- **Tight glycaemic control:**
  - Improved glycaemic control is associated with less diabetic retinopathy
  - There may be a transient worsening of the retinopathy in the first nine months of improved control
- **Treat other risk factors:**
  - Hypertension; hypercholesterolaemia; smoking cessation
  - Accelerated deterioration occurs in poor diabetic control, hypertension and pregnancy
- **VEGF inhibitor injections:**
  - Centre-involving (foveal) diabetic macular oedema > 400 microns (NICE approved)
  - Clinically significant macular oedema that is not centre involving is most likely to receive focal photocoagulation

- **Photocoagulation indications:**
  - ○ Maculopathy
  - ○ Proliferative diabetic retinopathy
- Pan-retinal photocoagulation prevents the ischaemic retinal cells secreting angiogenesis factors causing neovascularization
- Focal photocoagulation targets areas of leakage

COMPLICATIONS OF PROLIFERATIVE DIABETIC RETINOPATHY
- Vitreous haemorrhage (may require vitrectomy)
- Traction retinal detachment
- Neovascular glaucoma due to rubeosis iridis

Cataracts

CLINICAL SIGNS
- Loss of the red reflex – when a cataract is mature
- Cloudy lens or dark spokes with cortical cataract
- Associations: dystrophia myotonica (bilateral ptosis)

CAUSES
- Congenital (pre-senile): rubella, Turner's syndrome
- Acquired: **age** (usually bilateral), diabetes, drugs (steroids), radiation exposure, trauma and storage disorders

TREATMENT
- Surgery (outpatient):
  - ○ Phacoemulsification with prosthetic lens implantation
  - ○ Yttrium aluminium garnet (YAG) laser capsulotomy (if posterior capsular thickening post cataract operation)

Hyperthyroidism and Graves' disease
Please assess this 37-year-old female who has noticed weight loss, palpitations and a tremor.

History
GOITRE
- Usually non-tender (tender = thyroiditis)

THYROID STATUS
- Graves' disease patients may be hyperthyroid, euthyroid or hypothyroid depending on their stage of treatment
- Enquire about symptoms of hyperthyroidism:

Anxiety, restlessness, irritability	Heat intolerance	Tremor
Insomnia	Excess sweating	Palpitations
Impaired concentration	Increased appetite	Pruritis
	Weight loss	

EYE PROBLEMS
- See below; eye(s) may be painful

Examination
- **Smooth, diffuse goitre** with possible bruit (increased blood flow)
- No associated cervical lymphadenopathy

	Specific to Graves'	Hyperthyroidism
Eye signs	Proptosis	Lid retraction
	Chemosis	Lid lag
	Exposure keratitis	
	Ophthalmoplegia	
Peripheral signs	Thyroid acropachy	Agitation
	Pretibial myxoedema	Sweating
		Tremor
		Palmar erythema
		Sinus tachycardia/AF
		Brisk reflexes
		Hypertension
		Proximal myopathy

- Keratitis due to poor eye closure
- Optic nerve compression: loss of colour vision initially, then development of a central scotoma and reduced visual acuity
- Papilloedema may occur

Discussion

INVESTIGATION
- Thyroid function tests: TSH and T_3/T_4
- Thyroid autoantibodies
- Radioisotope scanning: increased uptake of I^{131} in Graves' disease, reduced in thyroiditis

TREATMENT
- β-Blocker, e.g. propranolol – symptom relief
- Carbimazole or propylthiouracil (both thionamides)
  - **Block and replace** with thyroxine
  - **Titrate** dose and monitor endogenous thyroxine
    - Stop at 18 months and assess for return of thyrotoxicosis; one-third of patients will remain euthyroid
- If thyrotoxicosis returns, the options are:
  - A repeat course of a thionamide
  - Radioiodine (I^{131}): hypothyroidism common
  - Subtotal thyroidectomy
- Severe ophthalmopathy may require high-dose steroids, orbital irradiation or surgical decompression to prevent visual loss
- **NOSPECS** mnemonic for the progression of eye signs in Graves' disease:
  - **N**o signs or symptoms
  - **O**nly lid lag/retraction
  - **S**oft tissue involvement
  - **P**roptosis
  - **E**xtraocular muscle involvement
  - **C**hemosis
  - **S**ight loss due to optic nerve compression and atrophy

Hypothyroidism

This 64-year-old female patient has been complaining of feeling the cold and has no energy.

History

SYMPTOMS

- Tired and low energy levels
- Cold intolerance
- Weight gain
- Constipation
- Hair loss, brittle nails, oedema
- Oligo- or amenorrhoea in women
- Decreased libido and erectile dysfunction in men
- Mental slowing → cognitive impairment

DRUG HISTORY

- Amiodarone, lithium and anti-thyroid drugs

ASSOCIATED ILLNESSES

- Previously treated thyroid disease
- Autoimmune: Addison's disease, vitiligo and T1DM
- Hypercholesterolaemia
- History of ischaemic heart disease: treatment with thyroxine may precipitate angina

Examination

- **Hands:**
  - ○ Slow pulse
  - ○ Dry skin
  - ○ Cool peripheries
- **Head/face/neck:**
  - ○ **'Peaches and cream'** complexion (anaemia and carotenaemia: thyroxine needed to convert carotene to vitamin A – thyroxine deficiency results in yellow/orange skin pigmentation)
  - ○ Eyes: **peri-orbital oedema, loss of eyebrows** and xanthelasma
  - ○ **Thinning hair**
  - ○ **Goitre or thyroidectomy scar**
- **Legs:**
  - ○ **Slow relaxing ankle jerk** (tested with patient kneeling on a chair)

COMPLICATIONS

- **Cardiac:** pericardial effusion (rub), congestive cardiac failure (oedema)
- **Neurological:** carpel tunnel syndrome (Phalen's/Tinel's test), proximal myopathy (difficulty stand from sitting) and ataxia

Discussion

INVESTIGATION

- **Blood:** TSH (↑ in thyroid failure, ↓ in pituitary failure), T_4 ↓, autoantibodies
- Associations: hyponatraemia, hypercholesterolaemia, macrocytic anaemia, consider short Synacthen test (exclude Addison's)
- **ECG:** pericardial effusion and ischaemia
- **CXR:** pericardial effusion and CCF

MANAGEMENT
- Thyroxine titrated to TSH suppression and clinical response
  - NB 1. Can precipitate angina
  - NB 2. Can unmask Addison's disease → crisis

CAUSES
- **Autoimmune:** Hashimoto's thyroiditis (+ goitre) and atrophic hypothyroidism
- **Iatrogenic:** post-thyroidectomy or I^{131}, amiodarone, lithium and anti-thyroid drugs
- **Iodine deficiency:** dietary ('Derbyshire neck')
- **Dyshormonogenesis**
- **Genetic:** Pendred's syndrome (with deafness)

Amenorrhoea
This 30-year-old nulliparous woman presents with amenorrhoea for four months and headaches, and had a car accident last month.

- **Diagnosis:** pituitary adenoma and multiple endocrine neoplasia (MEN) type 1
- **Differential diagnosis:** pregnancy, polycystic ovary syndrome (PCOS), premature ovarian failure, eating disorders, drug causes

History
- Confirm primary (never had a period) or **secondary amenorrhoea** (three or more missed periods in a previously menstruating female)
- If secondary:
  - Enquire about possibility of pregnancy
  - Enquire about extreme exercise, dietary changes and recent weight loss/gain
  - Hot or cold intolerance
  - **Headache**, fatigue, emotional stress
  - Ask about changes in vision – particularly **visual field loss**; near misses when driving the car; knocked over cups at home; walking into things
  - Any other hormone-related symptoms – loss of libido, excessive thirst (central diabetes insipidus), **galactorrhoea** (prolactinoma)
- Past medical history – gynae: endometriosis/PCOS, surgery/radiotherapy; renal stones and/or **parathyroidectomy** and thyroid disorders; indigestion/stomach ulcers
- Drug history – particularly antipsychotics (risperidone), but also chemotherapy, antidepressants (escitalopram, sertraline), treatments for endometriosis/fibrocystic breast (danazol)
- FH of malignancy/MEN 1 pedigree, premature menopause (ovarian failure)

Examination
- General inspection:
  - Spot diagnosis of acromegaly – large hands, prominent supra-orbital ridges, widely spaced teeth, macroglossia and prognathism
  - Subtotal/total parathyroidectomy scars, skin tumours – angiofibroma/lipoma
- Abdominal:
  - Laparotomy scars
  - Masses, hepatomegaly
- Neurology:
  - **Assess for visual field defects** – loss of peripheral vision (bitemporal hemianopia/bilateral superior quadrantanopia) due to compression of overlying nasal fibres decussating at optic chiasm

Discussion
INVESTIGATION
- Pregnancy test
- Blood test for endocrine abnormalities – prolactin, GH, PTH, Ca, TSH, T_4 and glucose
- Head CT/MRI to investigate for a pituitary adenoma

MANAGEMENT
- **Pituitary adenoma management:** observe (often benign), hormone (block and/or replace hormone secretion or shrink adenoma), radiotherapy, trans-sphenoidal surgery
- **MEN I treatments:**
  - **Medical:**
    - Hyperparathyroidism – calcimemetics, bisphosphonates
    - Prolactinoma – dopamine agonist (cabergoline)

- ○ GH-secreting adenoma – somatostatin analogues – octreotide
- ○ Gastrinoma – PPI/H2 blockers
- ○ **Surgery:**
  - ○ Subtotal/total parathyroidectomy
  - ○ Transsphenoidal pituitary adenoma/GEP tumour/adrenal tumour resection
- • Offer **genetic counselling**/screen first-degree relatives
- • Referral to a **fertility specialist** (for LH, FSH, GnRH tests) and genetic testing may be needed if a pituitary lesion has been ruled out

DIFFERENTIAL DIAGNOSIS
- • Causes of primary amenorrhoea
  - ○ Usually genetic. e.g. Turner's syndrome
- • Causes of secondary amenorrhoea – 6 Ps:
  - ○ Pregnancy
  - ○ Post-partum and breastfeeding
  - ○ Pills
  - ○ Premature menopause
  - ○ Polycystic ovary syndrome (causes 80% of anovulatory infertility)
  - ○ Pituitary adenoma (prolactinomas commonest)

MULTIPLE ENDOCRINE NEOPLASIA (MEN) 1
- • Inherited tumours: 1 in 30,000, autosomal dominant, *MEN1* gene, chromosome 11q13, 10% de novo mutation
  - ○ **P**arathyroid hyperplasia (90%)
  - ○ **P**ancreatic tumours (gastrinomas) (40–50%)
  - ○ **P**ituitary tumours (10–20%)
  - ○ Can also get other tumours of gastroenteropancreatic (GEP) tract: insulinoma, glucagonoma, VIP-secreting tumours; carcinoid, adrenal and skin tumours
- • **Tumour surveillance** with annual bloods and cross-sectional imaging every 5 years
- • Decreased life expectancy due to effects of malignancies: 50% survival at 50 years

TURNER'S SYNDROME
- • 1/2000 live births, usually diagnosed on karyotyping (45X).
- • Spot diagnosis – short stature, web neck, low-set ears and hair line, widely spaced nipples, absent secondary sexual characteristics (without HRT)
- • Usually managed in Turner's syndrome clinics due to multimorbidity: growth, sexual development, fertility (foetal germ cell apoptosis – streak ovaries) and psychological problems, deafness, diabetes mellitus, hypertension, ASD, bicuspid aortic valve and CoA
- • Cardiovascular morbidity shortens life expectancy by 10–15 years

Acromegaly
This 60-year-old male patient has been complaining of headaches.

History
HEADACHE
- Pituitary space-occupying lesion: early-morning headache, nausea
- Visual problems: tunnel vision (bitemporal hemianopia – noticeable when driving)
- Loss of libido and/or galactorrhoea

GENERAL OBSERVATIONS
- Change in appearance: photographs
- Tight-fitting jewellery
- Increase in size: shoes, gloves

ASSOCIATED CONDITIONS
- Diabetes mellitus

Examination: 'spot diagnosis'
- **Hands:** large 'spade like', **tight rings,*** coarse skin and **sweaty***
- **Face:** prominent supra-orbital ridges, prognathism, widely spaced teeth and macroglossia

COMPLICATIONS TO LOOK FOR: A, B, C . . .
- **A**canthosis nigricans
- **B**P ↑*
- **C**arpal tunnel syndrome
- **D**iabetes mellitus*
- **E**nlarged organs
- **F**ield defect*: bitemporal hemianopia
- **G**oitre, **g**astrointestinal malignancy
- **H**eart failure, **h**irsute, **h**ypopituitary
- **I**GF-1 ↑
- **J**oint arthropathy
- **K**yphosis
- **L**actation (galactorrhoea)
- **M**yopathy (proximal)

*Signs of active disease

Discussion
INVESTIGATIONS
- **Diagnostic**
  - Raised plasma **IGF-1**
  - **Non-suppression of growth hormone (GH)** after an oral glucose tolerance test (if IGF-1 level equivocal)
  - **MRI pituitary fossa:** pituitary adenoma
  - Also assess other pituitary functions
- **Complications**
  - **CXR:** cardiomegaly
  - **ECG:** ischaemia (DM and hypertension)
  - **Pituitary function tests:** TSH, ACTH, PRL and testosterone
  - **Glucose:** DM
  - **Visual perimetry:** bitemporal hemianopia
  - **Obstructive sleep apnoea** (in 50%): due to macroglossia

- Aim is to normalize GH and IGF-1 levels
- **Surgery:** trans-sphenoidal approach
  - ○ Medical post-op complications:
    - ○ Meningitis
    - ○ Diabetes insipidus
    - ○ Panhypopituitarism
- **Medical therapy:**
  - ○ Somatostatin analogues (octreotide – SC or IM depot), dopamine agonists (cabergoline – PO) block GH secretion
  - ○ GH receptor antagonists (pegvisomant – SC) block GH action
- **Radiotherapy** in non-surgical candidates

FOLLOW-UP
- Annual GH, prolactin, ECG, visual fields and MRI head

Causes of macroglossia
- **Acromegaly**
- Amyloidosis
- Hypothyroidism
- Down's syndrome

Acanthosis nigricans
- Brown 'velvet-like' skin change found commonly in the axillae
- Associations:
  - ○ Obesity
  - ○ Type II diabetes mellitus
  - ○ **Acromegaly**
  - ○ Cushing's syndrome
  - ○ Ethnicity: Indian subcontinent
  - ○ Malignancy, e.g. gastric carcinoma and lymphoma

Cushing's syndrome

This 44-year-old female patient has been gaining weight and has noticed difficulty in getting out of a chair.

History

SYMPTOMS
- Fatigue
- Easy bruising
- Weight gain
- Menstrual changes
- Loss of libido
- Acne
- Hirsutism
- Infections
- Depression
- Weakness (proximal myopathy)

DRUG HISTORY
- Exogenous vs endogenous steroid

ASSOCIATED PROBLEMS
- Visual problems: bitemporal hemianopia
- Skin hyperpigmentation
- Diabetes mellitus
- Hypertension

DIFFERENTIAL DIAGNOSIS
- Ethanol excess: pseudo-Cushing's

Examination

SPOT DIAGNOSIS
- **Face:** moon-shaped, red-faced, hirsute, with acne
- **Skin:** bruised, thin, with purple striae
- **Back:** 'buffalo hump'
- **Abdomen:** centripetal obesity
- **Legs:** wasting ('lemon on sticks' body shape) and oedema

COMPLICATIONS
- **Hypertension** (BP)
- **Diabetes mellitus** (random blood glucose)
- **Osteoporosis** (kyphosis)
- **Proximal myopathy** (ask the patient to cross their arms over their chest and stand up from a sitting position)

CAUSE
- **Exogenous:** signs of chronic condition (e.g. RA, COPD) requiring steroids
- **Endogenous:** bitemporal hemianopia and hyperpigmentation (if ACTH ↑)

Discussion
- **Cushing's disease:** glucocorticoid excess due to ACTH-secreting pituitary adenoma
- **Cushing's syndrome:** the physical signs of glucocorticoid excess

Causes of Cushing's syndrome

ACTH dependent	Cushing's disease (pituitary adenoma)
	Ectopic secretion of ACTH (non-pituitary tumour – e.g. bronchogenic carcinoma)
ACTH independent	Iatrogenic (exogenous steroids)
	Adrenocortical adenomas or carcinomas (secreting)

INVESTIGATION
- **Confirm high cortisol**
  - 24 h urinary collection for urinary free cortisol
  - Overnight dexamethasone suppression test (1 mg)
- **Suppressed cortisol:** alcohol/depression/obesity (pseudo-Cushing's)
- **If elevated cortisol confirmed, then identify cause:**
  - **ACTH level**
    - **High:** ectopic ACTH-secreting tumour or pituitary adenoma
    - **Low:** adrenal adenoma/carcinoma
  - **MRI pituitary fossa ± adrenal CT ± whole-body CT** to locate lesion
  - **Bilateral inferior petrosal sinus vein sampling** (best test to confirm pituitary vs ectopic origin; may also lateralize pituitary adenoma)
  - **High-dose dexamethasone suppression test may help identify cause:** cortisol will fall by >50% in those with ACTH-dependent Cushing's disease, but not where there is ectopic ACTH secretion or ACTH-independent adrenal adenoma or carcinoma

TREATMENT
- **Surgical:**
  - Trans-sphenoidal approach to remove pituitary tumours
  - Adrenalectomy for adrenal tumours
- **Nelson's syndrome:** bilateral adrenalectomy (scars) to treat Cushing's disease, causing massive production of ACTH (and melanocyte-stimulating hormone), due to lack of feedback inhibition, leading to hyper-pigmentation and pituitary overgrowth
- **Pituitary irradiation**
- **Medical:** Metyrapone

PROGNOSIS
- Untreated Cushing's syndrome: 50% mortality at 5 years (usually due to accelerated ischaemic heart disease secondary to diabetes and hypertension)

Causes of proximal myopathy
- **Inherited:**
  - Myotonic dystrophy
  - Muscular dystrophy
- **Endocrine:**
  - **Cushing's syndrome**
  - Hyperparathyroidism
  - Thyrotoxicosis
  - Diabetic amyotrophy

- **Inflammatory:**
  - Polymyositis
  - Rheumatoid arthritis
- **Metabolic:**
  - Osteomalacia
- **Malignancy:**
  - Paraneoplastic
  - Lambert–Eaton myasthenic syndrome
- **Drugs:**
  - Alcohol
  - Steroids

Addison's disease

Please assess this 59-year-old male patient; he was admitted as an emergency four days ago with postural hypotension and fatigue.

History
SYMPTOMS
- **Fatigue,** muscle weakness, low mood, loss of appetite, weight loss, **thirst (dehydration)**
- **Darkened skin** (Addison's disease)
- Fainting or cramps

CAUSE
- Known Addison's disease on steroid
- Other **autoimmune disease,** e.g. hypothyroidism, type I diabetes mellitus and vitiligo
- **TB or metastasis**

DIFFERENTIAL DIAGNOSIS
- Secondary adrenal insufficiency: pituitary adenoma or **sudden discontinuation of exogenous** steroid therapy

Examination
- Medic alert bracelet
- **Hyper-pigmentation:** palmar creases, scars, nipples and buccal mucosa
- **Postural hypotension**
- Visual fields: **bitemporal hemianopia** (pituitary adenoma)

CAUSE
- Signs of other associated autoimmune diseases
- Signs of TB or malignancy

Discussion
ADDISON'S DISEASE: PRIMARY ADRENAL INSUFFICIENCY
- Pigmentation due to a lack of feedback inhibition by cortisol on the pituitary, leading to raised ACTH and melanocyte-stimulating hormone
- In 80% of cases Addison's disease is due to an **autoimmune** process. Other causes include adrenal metastases, adrenal tuberculosis, amyloidosis, adrenalectomy and Waterhouse–Friderichsen syndrome (meningococcal sepsis and adrenal infarction)

INVESTIGATION ORDER
- **8 am cortisol:** no morning elevation suggests Addison's disease (unreliable)
- **Short Synacthen test:** cortisol fails to rise adequately (cortisol deficiency)
- **ACTH level** (>twofold elevation + cortisol deficiency = **primary adrenal insufficiency**)
- Measure aldosterone and renin to assess for concurrent mineralocorticoid deficiency
- **Adrenal imaging (primary) and/or pituitary imaging (secondary) with MRI or CT**

OTHER TESTS
- **Blood:** eosinophilia, ↓ Na^+ (kidney loss), ↑ K^+, ↑ urea (dehydration), ↓ glucose, adrenal autoantibodies (if autoimmune cause), thyroid function tests (hypothyroidism)
- **CXR:** malignancy or TB

TREATMENT
- **Acute (adrenal crisis)**
  - 0.9% saline **IV rehydration** +++ and glucose
  - **Hydrocortisone**
  - Treatment may unmask diabetes insipidus (cortisol is required to excrete a water load)
  - Anti-TB treatment increases the clearance of steroid, therefore higher doses required
- **Chronic**
  - **Education:** compliance, **increase steroid dose if 'ill'**, steroid card, medic alert bracelet
  - Titrate maintenance hydrocortisone (and fludrocortisone) dose to levels/response

PROGNOSIS
- Normal life expectancy

Index

Note: Page numbers with figures in *italic* and tables in **bold**.

abdominal discomfort 31, 83–85
abdominal examination 81–82
   chronic liver disease and hepatomegaly 83–85
   clinical mark sheet **80**
   haemochromatosis 86–87
   liver transplant patient 92
   renal enlargement 90–91
   renal patient 93–94
   splenomegaly 88–89
abdominal scars *92*
abnormal pupils 73
   Argyll Robertson pupil 74
   Holmes–Adie pupil 73–74
   Horner's pupil 73
   oculomotor (III) nerve palsy 74–75
   optic atrophy 75–76
acanthosis nigricans 204
accelerated phase hypertension 129
acromegaly 203–204
acute exacerbation treatment of COPD 9
acute pericarditis 124
acute pulmonary embolus 144–145
Addison's disease 208–209
adrenal insufficiency 208
advanced care planning 108–110
advanced decisions (directives) to refuse
    treatment (ADRT) 109–110, 112–113
age-related macular degeneration (AMD) 77
α1-antitrypsin deficiency 8
altered conscious state 135–136
amenorrhoea 201–202
amyotrophic lateral sclerosis 63
anaemia 151–152
angina (ischaemia) non-obstructive coronary
    artery (A(I)NOCA) 123
angina 22, 122–123
angioid streaks 176, 188
anhidrosis 73, 147
ankylosing spondylitis 185
anorexia nervosa 115
anterior ischaemic optic neuropathy 129
antibiotic prophylaxis 24
anti-muscle-specific-kinase (MuSK) 70
anti-nicotinic acetylcholine receptor (anti-AChR) 70

anti-phospholipid syndrome (APS) 181
anti-streptolysin O titre (ASOT) 28
anti-tachycardia pacing (ATP) 35
aortic incompetence (regurgitation) 25–26
aortic stenosis 22–24
aortic valve replacement 33
apical fibrosis 6
Argyll Robertson pupil 74
ascites 84
assessment order 99–100
asthma 172
   clinical consultations 142–143
   history taking 116–117
ataxia 131
   Friedreich's 42, 48, 50, 51, 59, 67, 76
   sensory 48
   vestibular 131
atrial fibrillation 125–126
atrial septal defect (ASD) 38
autoantibodies in liver disease 85
autoimmune hepatitis (AIH) 85
autosomal dominant polycystic kidney disease
    (ADPKD) 71, 90–91, 93, 94

back pain 185
bacterial endocarditis **29**, 149
bacterial meningitis 132
balloon aortic valvuloplasty (BAV) 23
Bamford classification of stroke 57
basal cell carcinoma 174
basal fibrosis 4
Bell's palsy 68
biventricular pacemakers 35
Blalock–Taussig shunts (BT shunts) 40
bloody diarrhoea 161
Bolam test 97
Bolitho test 97
bone pain 153–154
Bowen's disease 174
brain-stem death 113–115
brain stem reflexes 114
breaking bad news 96, 105
breathlessness 22
bronchial carcinoma, peripheral stigmata of 146

bronchiectasis 5
bronchoalveolar lavage 4

capacity 98–99, 106, 109–110, 113, 115
carcinoid syndrome 32
cardiac resynchronization therapy (CRT) 35
cardiopulmonary resuscitation (CPR) 103
cataracts 196
cell depletion therapy 180
cerebellar syndrome 53
Charcot joint 61
Charcot–Marie–tooth. *See* hereditary motor
    sensory neuropathy
chest pain:
    clinical consultations 122–123
    history taking 121, 124, 125, 127, 137, 146, 153
Child–Pugh classification of cirrhosis 84
chronic liver disease 10, 83–85
chronic obstructive airways disease (COPD) 8–9,
    119
chronic renal failure 10
chronic thromboembolic pulmonary hypertension
    (CTEPH) 145
cirrhosis 83, 84
closing click (CC) 33
cluster headache 132, 134
coarctation 40
coeliac disease 151–152
cogwheel rigidity 64
cold intolerance 201
collapsing pulse 20
colonic carcinoma 162
common law 97, 101, 106, 113
community-acquired pneumonia (CAP) 15
competency 98, 113
confidentiality 101, 111
congenital defects 38–39
congenital VSD, associations with 40
    coarctation 40
    Fallot's tetralogy 40
    heart failure 44–45
    hypertrophic (obstructive) cardiomyopathy
        42–43
    patent ductus arteriosus 40–41
congestive cardiac failure (CCF) 10
connective tissue disease 10, 30, 36
consent 98–99, 101, 113–115
    for blood sample 110
    for donor organs 45
    for insertion of chest drain 119
constrictive pericarditis 36–37
cord compression 59
coronary microcirculatory dysfunction (CMD) 123
cough:
    atrial septal defect 38

bronchiectasis 5
chest pain 122
dyspnoea 142, 144
haemoptysis 146
lung cancer 12
pericarditis 124
persistent fever 148
pneumonia 15, 139
respiratory examination 2
sign 2
surgical respiratory cases 7
syncope 137
systemic sclerosis 183
cranial nerves 47, *47*
Crohn's disease 161–162, **162**
CURB-65 score 15
Cushing's syndrome 205–207
cystic fibrosis 14

deep vein thrombosis (DVT) 166–167
defibrillators 35
diabetes mellitus (DM) 50
    and complications 191–192
    diabetic retinopathy 194–195
    haemochromatosis 86
    history taking 122, 131
    quaternary syphilis by 74
    renal patient 93–94
    skin complaints 192–193
diabetic education 115
diabetic ketoacidosis 115, 135
diabetic maculopathy *195*
diabetic retinopathy 194–196
diarrhoea, infectious:
    inflammatory bowel disease 161, 164–165
    triage into bloody and non-bloody **164**
dieting 115
difficult patients 106
disability 55, 106, 178
disease-modifying anti-rheumatoid drugs
    (DMARDs) 180
distal intestinal obstruction syndrome (DIOS) 14
dizziness:
    anaemia 153
    chronic hypoxaemia 130
    postural 140
    syncope 137
doctrine of double effect 102
donation after brain death (DBD) 114
donation after cardiac death (DCD) 114
donor cards 113
do not attempt cardiopulmonary resuscitation
    (DNA-CPR) orders 102
double lung transplant 7
double vision 54–55, 70

Driver and Vehicle Licensing Agency (DVLA) 101, 106–107, 138
driving restrictions **107**
drowsiness 135–136
Duckett–Jones diagnostic criteria 28
Duke's criteria for infective endocarditis 24
duty of candour 108
duty of care 97
dysarthria 51, 56
dyspnoea:
　acute pulmonary embolus 144–145
　aortic stenosis 22–24
　asthma 142–143
　consultations 142
　prosthetic valves 33–34
dystrophia myotonica 51–52

early diastolic murmur (EDM) *25*
Ebstein's anomaly 31
eczema 171–172
Ehlers–Danlos 176, 188
Eisenmenger's syndrome 130
ejection click (EC) 30, 127
ejection systolic murmur (ESM) *22, 32, 42*
empyema 10–11
end-of-life decisions 102–103
endocarditis 22, **25**
　bacterial **29**, 149
　Duke's criteria for 24
　infective 31, 34
endovascular aortic repair (EVAR) 40
enlarged nerves 72
enophthalmos 72
epilepsy **107**, 111, 138
EPIlepsy, LOw Intelligence, Adenoma sebaceum (EPILOIA) 71
eruptive xanthomata 190
erythema nodosum 172–173
ethics:
　competency and consent 98
　confidentiality 101
　end-of-life decisions 102–103
　legal aspects 98–100
　principles of medical ethics 97
euthanasia 103
extra-ocular muscle palsies 70
eyes:
　abnormal pupils 73
　age-related macular degeneration 77
　cataracts 196
　cranial nerves 47
　double vision 54, 70
　hyperthyroidism and Graves' disease 197–198
　multiple sclerosis 54
　old tuberculosis 6

optic atrophy 75
retinal artery occlusion 79
retinal pathology 77–79
retinitis pigmentosa 78
tuberous sclerosis 71
visual field defects *47*

fall and fragility fracture 141
Fallot's tetralogy. *See* tetralogy of Fallot (ToF)
family screening 87
fasciculations 48
fatigue 44–45, 148, 153, 208–209
fever:
　glandular 155–156
　persistent 148–150
　rheumatic 28
'fish-mouth' scars 176
fixed split-second heart sounds *38*
flank scar *93*
focal segmental glomerulosclerosis (FSGS) 158
Foster–Kennedy syndrome 76
frailty assessment 141
Friedreich's ataxia 42, 48, 50, 51, 59, 67, 76
fundoscopy 194
fundus 75–76

gastroenteropancreatic tract (GEP tract) 202
generalized seizure 111
giant cell arteritis 79
Gillick competent 98
glandular fever 155–156
gluten-sensitive enteropathy 151
goitre 197
Good Medical Practice (GMP) 96
gout 189
granuloma annulare 193
granulomatous polyarteritis 9
Graves' disease 197–198
growth hormone (GH) 203
gum hypertrophy 92
gynaecomastia 85

haemochromatosis 86–87
haemoptysis 146–147
handicap 55, 178
headache:
　acromegaly 203
　clinical consultations 132–134
　cluster 132, 134
　medication overuse 133
　migrainous 132
　tension 132, 134
　thunderclap 132, 134
heart failure 44–45
Henoch–Schönlein purpura 173

hepatocellular carcinoma (HCC) 86
hepatomegaly 83–85
hereditary haemorrhagic telangiectasia (HHT)
    2, 152
hereditary motor sensory neuropathy (HMSN) 66
Holmes–Adie pupil 73, 73–74
Horner's pupil 73, 73
Human Organ Transplant Act (1989) 114
Human Tissue Act (1961) 114
Huntington's chorea 111–112
hypercalcaemia 191
hypercholesterolaemia 193
hyperextensible joints 176–177
hyperparathyroidism 191
hypertension 127–129
    pulmonary 17–18, 22, 27
    renal enlargement 90–91
hypertriglyceridaemia 193
hypertrophic (obstructive) cardiomyopathy
    42–43
hypothyroidism 199–200

Iliac fossa scar 93
immunomodulation therapy 180
immunosuppression 4
immunosuppressive medication 92
impairment 55
implantable cardiac defibrillators (ICD) 35
implied consent 98, 113
infection:
    endocarditis 24, 29, 31, 34, 149
    persistent fever 148
    pneumonia 15–16
    splenomegaly 88–89, 89
inflammatory bowel disease (IBD) 159, 161–163
information delivery 104, 119
internuclear ophthalmoplegia 54, 54
invasive coronary angiography 123
Ipsilateral Horner's syndrome 147
iron deficiency anaemia 81
irritable bowel syndrome (IBS) 161
ischaemic heart disease (IHD) 119

jaundice 159–160
Jugular venous pressure waves (JVP waves) 5, 17,
    20, 36, 36
justice 97

Kernig's sign 133
ketoacidosis 135
kidney–pancreas transplantation 93–94
Koebner phenomenon 171

lacunar anterior circulation stroke (LACS) 57
Lambert–Eaton myasthenic syndrome (LEMS) 70

lasting power of attorney 99, 112
lateral medullary syndrome 57
lateral thoracotomy 33
law:
    advanced decisions to refuse treatment
        109–110
    best interests of patient 99
    competency, capacity and consent 98
    end-of-life decisions 102–103
    in medicine 97–103
    medico-legal system 97
    negligence 97
leg oedema 157–158
leg ulcers 168–169
lethargy. See fatigue
Lhermitte's sign 55
liver function tests (LFT) 6, 160
liver transplant patient 92
lobectomy 7
long-term oxygen therapy (LTOT) 8, 9
loud first heart sound opening snap (OS) 27
lower limb dermatomes 60
lower motor neurone (LMN) 47
lung biopsy 4
lung cancer 12–13
lung disease 17
lung function tests 4, 12
lupus pernio 173
Lyme disease 138
lymphadenopathy 88
    cervical 81, 197
    feel femoral pulses and assess for 82
    glandular fever 155–156
lymphoma 36–37

macroglossia 204
maculopathy 194–195
malaise 12–13
malignancy:
    abdominal examination 84
    active incurable malignancy 45
    cholangiocarcinoma 159
    haemoptysis 146
    hypercalcaemia 191
    skin malignancy 92, 174–175
malignant hyperpyrexia syndrome 148
malignant hypertension 129
malignant melanoma 175
Marcus–Gunn pupil 75
Marfan's syndrome 186–187
mastectomy scars 3
medial longitudinal fasciculus (MLF) 54
medical ethics. See ethics
medication overuse headache 133
medico-legal system 97

meningitis 134
meningococcal meningitis 133
Mental Capacity Act (2005) 99
Mental Health Act (1983) 99, 113, 115
mesothelioma 11
metastases 146, 174
mid-diastolic murmur (MDM) *25, 27*
midline sternotomy 33
migrainous headache 132
mitral incompetence 29–30
mitral stenosis 27–28
mitral valve prolapse (MVP) 42
mitral valve replacement *33*
mobility:
    ankylosing spondylitis 185
    syncope 139–140
monoclonal antibodies 134
mononeuritis multiplex 50
motor neurone disease (MND) 63
multiple drusen *77*
multiple endocrine neoplasia (MEN)
        129, 201, 202
multiple sclerosis 54–55, 119, 129, 131
multisystem atrophy (MSA) 64, 138
murmur 20, 25, 30, 32, 122, 130, 149, 186
muscle wasting 51, 178
myasthenia gravis 70
myocardial infarction (MI) 119
myotonia 51
myotonic pupil. *See* Holmes–Adie pupil

nail pitting 171
necrobiosis lipoidica diabeticorum 192, 193
negligence 97, 108
Nelson's syndrome 206
neovascularization of the (optic) disc (NVD) *195*
nephrectomy *93*
nephrotic syndrome 157–158
neurofibromatosis 72
neuropathic arthropathy 61
neuropathic leg ulcer 168
new vessels elsewhere (NVE) *195*
night vision 78
nodules 173
non-compliant diabetic 115
non-compliant patient 106
non-maleficence 97
non-small cell lung cancer (NSCLC) 12, 13, 147
Noonan's syndrome 32
numbness 185, 188

obesity 189
occupational therapy 55
oculomotor (III) nerve palsy 74–75

old tuberculosis 6
opening click (OC) 33
opening snap (OS) *27*
optic atrophy 75–76
optic disc swelling 129
organ donation 113–115
organ donation law in UK 114–115
orthostatic hypotension 138
Osler–Weber–Rendu syndrome 152
osteoarthritis 189–190. *See also* rheumatoid
        arthritis
osteoporotic risk assessment 141
overdose 112–113

pacemakers 35, 78
Paget's disease 76, 188
palliative care 13, 103, 109
palmar erythema 84
palpitations 38, 42–43, 125–126, 197–198
pan-systolic murmur (PSM) *29–31*
Pancoast's tumour 147
papillitis/optic neuritis 129
papilloedema 129
papules 173
paracetamol overdose 112–113
paraesthesia 125–126
Parkinson's disease 64–65
partial anterior circulation stroke (PACS) 57
patent ductus arteriosus (PDA) 40–41
percussion myotonia 51
percutaneous pulmonary valve implantation
        (PPVI) 32
pericarditis with effusion 124
peripheral neuropathy 59, 72, 168
persistent cough 5
persistent fever 148–150
phrenic nerve crush 6
physiotherapy 5, 14
pleural aspiration 10
pleural effusion 10–11
plombage 6
pneumonectomy 7
pneumonia 15–16
pneumothorax 119, 142, 143
polycystic ovary syndrome (PCOS) 201
post-exposure prophylaxis (PEP) 110
posterior inferior cerebellar artery (PICA) 57
post lung transplant 9
postural dizziness 140
postural hypotension 208–209
Potts shunt 40
pregnancy:
    epilepsy 111
    hypertension 127–128

multiple sclerosis 54–55
  palmar erythema 84
  secondary amenorrhoea 202
primary biliary cirrhosis (PBC) 85
primary lateral sclerosis 63
primary progressive MS (PPMS) 54
primary sclerosing cholangitis (PSC) 85, 163
productive cough 15–16
progressive bulbar palsy 63
progressive spinal muscular atrophy 63
progressive supranuclear palsy 64
proliferative diabetic retinopathy 196
prosthetic valves 33–34
  aortic valve replacement *33*
  mitral valve replacement *33*
  scars on inspection *33*
proximal myopathy 206
pseudoxanthoma elasticum 176
psoriasis 170–171
psychosocial issues 170
ptosis **52**, 72
public law 97
pulmonary arterial hypertension (PAH) 17
pulmonary embolism (PE) 117–118
pulmonary fibrosis 4
pulmonary hypertension 17–18
pulmonary stenosis 32
pulmonary vasculitis 2
purpura 173

radiotherapy 3, 12, 13, 36–37
rapid antigen detection test (RADT) 28
rashes. *See* red rashes
Raynaud's phenomenon 181, 183
Recommended Summary Plan for Emergency
  Care and Treatment process (ReSPECT
  process) 102–103
red rashes 170–173
  eczema 171–172
  erythema nodosum 172–173
  Henoch–Schönlein purpura 173
  psoriasis 170–171
  systemic lupus erythematosus 181–182
refractory angina 123
relapsing-remitting MS (RRMS) 54
relative afferent pupillary defect (RAPD) 75
renal enlargement 90–91
renal transplant patient 93–94
retinal artery occlusion 79
retinal pathology 77
  age-related macular degeneration 77
  retinal artery occlusion 79
  retinal vein occlusion 79
  retinitis pigmentosa 78

retinal vein occlusion 79
retinitis pigmentosa 78, *78*
retinopathy, diabetic 194–196
rheumatic fever 28
rheumatoid arthritis (RA) 9, 178–180
Romberg's test 140

sabre tibia 188, **188**
Saccharine ciliary motility test 5
sanctity of life 102
scar:
  Ehlers–Danlos 176, 188
  haemochromatosis 86
  liver transplant patient 92
  neurofibromatosis 72
  renal patient 93
  thoracotomy 7
scleroderma 2
secondary amenorrhoea 201
secondary hyperlipidaemia 193
secondary progressive MS (SPMS) 54
seizures 71, 138
self-discharging patient 106
sensory ataxia 48
shared decision making 117–118
shortness of breath. *See* dyspnoea
sickle cell disease 153–154
single lung transplant 7
Sjögren's syndrome 181
skin. *See also* rashes
  diabetes and 192–193
  Henoch–Schönlein purpura 173
  hyperextensible joints 176–177
  malignancy 174–175
  psoriasis 170–171
  systemic lupus erythematosus 181–182
  tuberous sclerosis 71
small cell lung carcinoma (SCLC) 12, 13, 147
small pupil 72
spastic legs 59–60
spinal cord lesion 59–60
splenomegaly 88–89, **89**
squamous cell carcinoma 174–175
statute law 97, 114
stigmata 93
  of bronchial carcinoma 146
  of chronic liver disease 88
  immunosuppressant 90
  of venous hypertension 168
stroke 56–58
  Bamford classification of 57
  brainstem structures affected by right-sided
    lesion *57*
  clinical consequences of lesion **58**

subcutaneous implantable cardiac defibrillators (S-ICD) 35
supraclavicular lymphadenopathy 147
surgical respiratory cases 7
surgical valve replacement, choice of **34**
Surveillance, Epidemiology and End Results (SEER) 13
swollen ankles 32
swollen calf 166–167
swollen hands 183–184
syncope 22, 137–138
syringomyelia 61–62
systemic lupus erythematosus (SLE) 181–182
systemic sclerosis 183–184

tension headache 132, 134
tertiary syphilis 76
tetralogy of Fallot (ToF) 32, 40
thoracoplasty 6
thrombolysis in myocardial infarction (TIMI) risk score 123
thunderclap headache 132, 134
thyroid 125, 197
tiredness. See fatigue
tort law 97
total anterior circulation stroke (TACS) 57
transcatheter edge-to-edge repair (TEER) 30
transcutaneous aortic valve implantation (TAVI) 23
transient ischaemic attack (TIA) 56
transjugular intrahepatic portosystemic shunt (TIPS) 32
transvenous implantable cardiac defibrillators (TV-ICD) 35
traveller's diarrhoea. See diarrhoea, infectious
treatment order 100
tremor 64–65
trespass 97
tricuspid incompetence 31
trigeminal neuralgia 133
tuberculosis 6
tuberous sclerosis 71
tunnel vision 78, 137, 203

ulcerative colitis (UC) 119, **162**
upper-limb dermatomes 62

upper motor neurone (UMN) 47
urinary tract infection (UTI) 139
Uthoff's phenomenon 55

vaccination compliance 116–117
valve replacement 33
venous leg ulcer 168–169
ventricular interdependence 37
ventricular septal defect 39
vestibular ataxia 131
visual evoked potentials (VEPs) 55
visual field defects 47, 47, 201
vitamin K 160

walking problems 59–60, 64–65, 131
Wallenberg syndrome. See lateral medullary syndrome
warfarin **34**, 108, 137
Waterston shunt 40
weakness:
  Cushing's syndrome 205
  dystrophia myotonica 51
  facial 68–69
  hereditary motor sensory neuropathy 66
  motor neurone disease 63
  multiple sclerosis 54
  syringomyelia 61
weight gain 36–37, 115
weight loss:
  chronic liver disease and hepatomegaly 83
  inflammatory bowel disease 161
  lung cancer 12
  surgical respiratory cases 7
Wells' criteria 144
wheezing:
  bronchiectasis 5
  carcinoid syndrome 32
  chronic obstructive airways disease 8, 9
  cystic fibrosis 14
  dyspnoea 142
  polyphonic 172
Wilson's disease 131
withdrawing/withholding treatment 102
worsening mobility 139–140

xanthomata 193